LOVE BETS

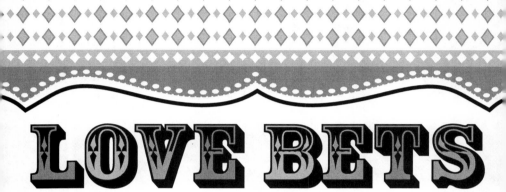

LOVE BETS

300 WAGERS TO SPICE UP YOUR LOVE LIFE

SHARON NAYLOR

Adams Media
New York London Toronto Sydney New Delhi

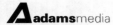

Adams Media
An Imprint of Simon & Schuster, Inc.
57 Littlefield Street
Avon, Massachusetts 02322

For information about special discounts for bulk purchases, please contact Simon & Schuster Special Sales at 1-866-506-1949 or business@simonandschuster.com.

The Simon & Schuster Speakers Bureau can bring authors to your live event. For more information or to book an event contact the Simon & Schuster Speakers Bureau at 1-866-248-3049 or visit our website at www.simonspeakers.com.

Interior illustration © rudi ornetsmüller / istockphoto.com.

Manufactured in the United States of America

10 9 8 7 6 5 4 3 2 1

Library of Congress Cataloging-in-Publication Data has been applied for.

ISBN 978-1-5986-9577-9

FOR JOE

CONTENTS

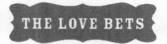

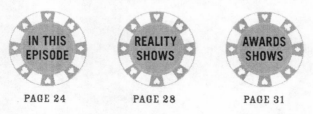

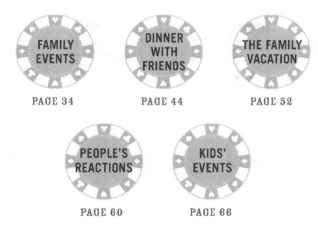
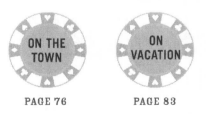

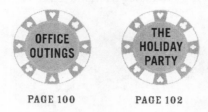
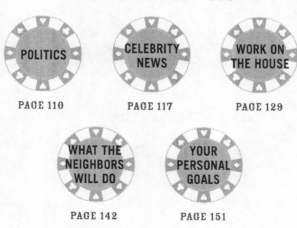

THE WAGERS

INTRODUCTION

The couple that plays together stays together.

Look in any "how to keep your relationship strong" book or article, and you'll see plenty of advice on "keeping things fun" and "spicing up your love life." Novelty is a key ingredient in a healthy love life, and so is laughter. Plenty of it. Sharing experiences and interests also rank high on the relationship longevity list, whether you're in a fresh, new relationship, a longtime dating relationship, engaged, newly married, or married *forever*.

So where do you get all this novelty, laughter, shared experiences, and spiciness? From making romantic wagers! As a couple, you'll bet on everything from the outcome of the Super Bowl to who gets voted off *American Idol* to who gets drunk and sloppy at the company holiday party. I've collected 300 different wagers for you both to use over time, in any situation from sporting events to vacations to lazy Sundays when you have absolutely nothing going on. And if you're partnered with a sports fan, this wager plan is a great way to share his or her favorite pastime in a whole new way.

Romantic wagers can bring new life to the things you share together as a couple. They can also get you through some of the less pleasant things in life like the annual, required family vacation or a five-hour drive to one of your friends' weddings. Or a dinner party at his mother's house. That way, you can walk into his mother's tension-filled obligatory dinner party knowing that you have a bet on whether or not she'll mention one of his ex-girlfriends. When she does, instead of fuming, you know that you have a box of Godiva chocolates coming to you. The bet allows you both to laugh off the social gaffe instead of fighting about it. Romantic wagers, then, can add humor to the minefields of your social and family obligations.

If you'd like your partner to get involved in the activities you love, but you just haven't found a way to entice him or her, perhaps a few romantic wagers will add that element of friendly competition that will engage interest. For that art exhibit you'd like to attend, the wager might be: If there's a canvas that displays a female nude, I will pose nude for you as you draw or paint a likeness of me—no photographs allowed. That, and the fact that there will be free wine and snacks at the gallery should add a new dimension to your night out.

Of course, romantic wagers are just for fun. They are never to be used to manipulate your partner, make them uncomfortable, humiliate them, or prey on a weakness or insecurity. They're also *not* for financial gain. This isn't gambling we're endorsing here, and at no time should a wager be: You'll pay off my Visa bill. I've collected hundreds of tame, romantic, and racy wager payouts for you to consider, and there's space at the back of this book for you both to record your own ideas. And it's a rule of this book that either player can veto any suggested bet or wager. You're not adversaries, trying to get something out of your partner through a crafty twisting of a fun game; you're introducing *Love Bets* into your everyday routines, special events, and outings as a way to add a fresh level of enjoyment to your relationship. Through them, you'll be reminded of your partner's adventurous, daring, or silly side, an impressive skill in cooking or artistry, and yes, a sexy side that you might not have seen or acknowledged much in the recent past.

Romantic wagers wake you both up to the many different facets of your personalities, through play and delicious anticipation, creativity, and the relationship-enhancing bonus benefit of displaying integrity. You made the bet, you keep it.

You're also showing your partner how much you care by crafting personalized bets and wagers that reflect your knowledge and love of the person you're involved with.

And of course, if you're not in a committed relationship right now, but are in a place in your life where you're going on first, second, or third dates, even blind dates, where conversation can get a little awkward at times, specially selected romantic wagers can break the ice, show your personality, and even better, reveal your date's personality. If he cringes at the idea of making a little wager on something going on around you—name the next song the cover band plays—then you know he doesn't share your same playful nature. If you're hitting it off, the romantic wager game can go on for hours . . . and often becomes one of those things that carries on through your next few dates as a way to play, laugh, challenge each other, and enjoy the date even more.

So now you know what this book can bring into your relationship, and that you can customize the level of romantic or racy wagers you have in mind. But I also encourage you to write in this book and make it a keepsake of the wagers you make with each other. Underneath each bet, write down the date and any details about how you used it, who won, and what you wagered. Doing so makes this book a keepsake of your relationship, something to look back through on an anniversary and relive your playful pastime and saucy suggestions. The written record can up the ante on your love life by challenging you to get even more creative, even sexier or more indulgent with your wagers, repeat your favorite bets, and even pull you out of any months-long ruts where you've both been too busy with work and stress to really connect. "Hey, remember this book? Remember when we went to the art gallery? Let's start doing these again."

Then you're back to adventure, novelty, creativity, and surprising each other with your personalized wager deliveries. You'll be laughing together again in no time, and someone's going to be washing some-one else's car with their shirt off really soon. Which could inspire another wager: How long until the neighbors call the cops? Just kidding—no wager should ever put you in danger or break a law. (Are you listening, those of you who are thinking, "Sex in public places!"?) Racy is always way better than raunchy, and the last thing I want as a result of this book is photos on the Internet that would prevent you from running for public office someday.

Make this book a keepsake of all the fun, romantic, and racy wagers you've made with one another. Include the date, where you were, what the bet was, and who won. Get ready to play together and stay together for a long, long time to come!

THE LOVE BETS

PART 1
SPORTS
AND COMPETITION

Whether you're competing against one another in a game of tennis, mini golf, one-on-one basketball, or watching the big game on television or in a stadium, you can turn your competitive edge into a romantic wager. What better incentive to make that three-pointer or sink that hole-in-one than knowing that you could win a massage at home later?

IT'S YOU VERSUS ME

PAGE 4

ON THE BIG SCREEN

PAGE 6

AT THE STADIUM

PAGE 15

LOVE BET #1

Who will be the winner of this game of [whatever sport we're playing]?

IT'S YOU VERSUS ME

If it's a back-and-forth competition where you're ahead first, then he catches up, then you take over the lead, that adds to the adrenaline and excitement levels. May the best man or woman win.

THE WINNER GETS	....
WHO WON?	....
DATE	....
SPECIAL PROVISIONS	....

LOVE BET #2

Who will be the winner half-way through this game we're playing?

In bowling, that would be the fifth frame. In racquetball, you can set a time limit of a half hour with your watch set to beep at the winning moment, and so on. Rather than have one bet going, you can turn this fun date into a collection of bets, with wagers won several times during play. You might even break it down further, with the winner of every quarter or the winner of each hole during mini golf. So if you have a great hole or frame, you become a winner, too. This levels the playing field, and both men and women who dominate in whatever game they're playing say they'd rather have multiple bets going so that they're not dominating their date to the point of frustration and greed.

THE WINNER GETS	....
WHO WON?	....
DATE	....
SPECIAL PROVISIONS	....

LOVE BET #3

Who will be the first one to make that special play?

You know, the big play that takes fantastic skill—or pure, dumb luck—like a hole-in-one, birdie, 3-point shot, sinking two balls at once in a game of pool, a bull's-eye in darts, and so on. At the start of your competitive date, you'll name that special shot as a shared goal within your winner bet, perhaps: Whoever gets a hole-in-one wins [wager.] It might happen during your game, or it might happen the next time you play (which is a great way to ask for a second date!), so you can carry that wager over to the next game.

THE WINNER GETS	....
WHO WON?	....
DATE	....
SPECIAL PROVISIONS	....

LOVE BET #4

Who will be the first one to make the big mistake?

If you're the types who are able to poke fun at yourselves and at each other without taking competition too seriously, then this bet is for you. Some people get really mad at themselves if their golf ball lands in a sand trap or if they get a gutter ball in bowling, an air ball in basketball, and so on. They turn beet red and get angry, and then the game (and thus the date) is no fun at all. Same goes for the partner who likes to tease mercilessly about any mistakes made. "You stink at this game!" is neither loving nor romantic. So make this wager only if you know that you can laugh together when you make a bad play.

THE WINNER GETS	....
WHO WON?	....
DATE	....
SPECIAL PROVISIONS	....

IT'S YOU VERSUS ME ◀ 5

LOVE BET #5

For football, who will win the coin toss?

ON THE BIG SCREEN

If you're not familiar with the sport, the coin-toss winner decides if they will kick off or receive the ball, and in big football games like the Super Bowl, they usually invite Hall of Famers or other notable people to participate. You can make this bet ahead of time, or one of you can call it when the coin is in the air.

THE WINNER GETS	....
WHO WON?	....
DATE	....
SPECIAL PROVISIONS	....

LOVE BET #6

For football, will your team decide to receive or kick?

Since they almost always decide to receive, to get the first shot at scoring, make sure you choose Receive. Even if you have very little knowledge of football, you'll impress your date by knowing this tidbit about the game.

THE WINNER GETS	....
WHO WON?	....
DATE	....
SPECIAL PROVISIONS	....

LOVE BET #7

For football, which side of the field will that team request?

Here's another opportunity to impress your all-about-the-game date. If the stadium is not a dome, and the field is open to the elements, the wind plays a big factor in which side of the field a team will choose. The wind affects passes, kickoffs, and field goal attempts, so make sure you listen to the commentators for any mention of which way the wind is blowing. And take a look at the flags flying on top of the open-air stadium—they'll be flapping with the wind, so score points with your date by saying, "Wait, I need to see how the wind is at the stadium."

THE WINNER GETS	
WHO WON?	
DATE	
SPECIAL PROVISIONS	

LOVE BET #8

For football, which side of the television screen will the first score—touchdown, field goal, or safety—be shown on?

This is a "Right" or "Left" answer most of the time, but be aware that you can say "Neither" for instances where a field goal attempt is filmed from behind the field goal. That score might be in the center of your television screen, so if you like the adrenaline rush of slim odds, wager big on your risky Neither bet!

THE WINNER GETS	
WHO WON?	
DATE	
SPECIAL PROVISIONS	

LOVE BET #9

For football, will the first cheerleader shown after the kickoff be a blonde, brunette, or redhead?

The camera loves the beautiful women on the sidelines, and the game has to get great ratings, so the network almost always cuts to a shot of a cheerleader. This is a quick, early-in-the-game bet that can get your wagers in action before any end-of-game score bets, and it's purely a chance bet, which can give you better odds of winning than bets where you need an in-depth knowledge of the game. Specify that the cheerleader in question has to have her own shot, not be part of a group of cheerleaders. Your bet holds until the next shot of a cheerleader solo.

THE WINNER GETS ....

WHO WON? ....

DATE ....

SPECIAL PROVISIONS ....

LOVE BET #10

The first commercial after kickoff will be for which kind of product?

Think soda, beer, car, erectile-dysfunction medication, and so on. For an extra add-on to the wager, write down the brand name of that product. And you have to be specific, such as Bud Light rather than Budweiser.

THE WINNER GETS ....

WHO WON? ....

DATE ....

SPECIAL PROVISIONS ....

Who will be the first celebrity shown in attendance at the big game?

While the camera loves cheerleaders, it also loves celebrities in attendance at the game. So you can have a little fun with audience shots by guessing which stars will be shown. It helps if you know the "usuals" who are shown often at games (which will impress your date!). For instance, if you're watching a Red Sox game, the odds are good that you'll see Ben Affleck and Jennifer Garner. If you're watching a Nets game, you may see Jay Z (who's a part owner of the team) and Beyoncé.

THE WINNER GETS	....
WHO WON?	....
DATE	....
SPECIAL PROVISIONS	....

What will the first score be?

For football, will it be a touchdown? Field goal? Safety? For basketball, will it be a layup or a three-pointer? Here is a chance to show off your knowledge of the game, and it starts off your viewing with a little bit of chancy excitement.

THE WINNER GETS	....
WHO WON?	....
DATE	....
SPECIAL PROVISIONS	....

In basketball, who will make the first dunk?

If you're not familiar with the playing styles of the team members, ask your date for a list of three of the players who often dunk. Then you choose from one of them. And if you want to add an extra layer of fun to this bet, specify that the player has to hang from the rim for a second or add a second wager to the bet if he or she does.

THE WINNER GETS	....
WHO WON?	....
DATE	....
SPECIAL PROVISIONS	....

Will there be a bench-clearing brawl?

This one is best for baseball games, especially when the teams are bitter rivals, although basketball games have been known to feature some bench-clearers. Yes, it's mildly evil to bet on violence, but this is a fun extra bet to have going when you're betting on game scores and MVPs. It doesn't happen often, so this is a fun long shot bet.

THE WINNER GETS	....
WHO WON?	....
DATE	....
SPECIAL PROVISIONS	....

Will anyone be ejected from the game?

It takes some pretty bad sportsmanship, but it has been happening more often in games from all sports. Referees and umpires take player safety and decency pretty seriously now, so you will see a "You're outta here!" gesture when a player crosses the line. As a wager doubler, name the player most likely to be ejected from the game, and don't forget that coaches have been tossed as well.

THE WINNER GETS ....

WHO WON? ....

DATE ....

SPECIAL PROVISIONS ....

Name the winner of the game when the score is close.

When it's a close game, it gets very exciting at the end, especially if the play goes into overtime and it all comes down to one kick or one batter in extra innings. While all the other fans are hoping for a win to boost the team record, you're hoping for a win to get that wager the two of you have. It all just increases the thrill of watching the game together.

THE WINNER GETS ....

WHO WON? ....

DATE ....

SPECIAL PROVISIONS ....

Will the point difference in the final score be more than ten points?

It's not a blowout, per se, but you're betting on a double-digit win. And when there's a comeback at the end of the game with not enough time for your team to actually win, you win if they get within ten points of the other team's lead. So this is a great secondary bet in addition to who will win.

THE WINNER GETS ....

WHO WON? ....

DATE ....

SPECIAL PROVISIONS ....

What color Gatorade will be dumped on the coach at the end of the game?

This longtime tradition in playoff and championship games always seems to catch the coaches by surprise. Hard to believe they don't know it's coming! Gatorade only gets dumped on the coach for championship and playoff games, so don't take this sucker bet for regular-season games.

THE WINNER GETS ....

WHO WON? ....

DATE ....

SPECIAL PROVISIONS ....

Name the MVP of the game.

If you're a true newbie to sports, MVP stands for Most Valuable Player. You might think it's always going to be the quarterback in the Super Bowl, but it's often the player who got the most yardage or set a record for scoring or was pivotal in the win through a series of big plays. Again, ask your partner to list three or four likely players for you to choose from if you're not familiar with the team members, or go online before the game starts to check out their stats. Your partner might love researching with you.

THE WINNER GETS ....
WHO WON? ....
DATE ....
SPECIAL PROVISIONS ....

For tennis, what color outfit will [player] be wearing?

Tennis has become a fashion sport, with the Williams sisters leading the way in pleather and miniskirts. If you're about to watch hours of tennis, make it a sport of your own by guessing the color of outfits worn by both male and female players.

THE WINNER GETS ....
WHO WON? ....
DATE ....
SPECIAL PROVISIONS ....

Name a song that will be played in the stadium, that you can hear during the broadcast or before a commercial break.

Pull out that stadium music CD, and make sure it's a current one so that you get the best selection of songs that are being played now. "Take Me Out to the Ballgame" is almost always heard at baseball games and the "Cha Cha Slide" is almost always heard at minor league baseball games. You can narrow this bet to the first song heard, so that you're not a slave to the television set the whole night, or so that listening for songs at the stadium doesn't become a job.

THE WINNER GETS	....
WHO WON?	....
DATE	....
SPECIAL PROVISIONS	....

For baseball, which player will be the first to hit a home run?

Hopefully, your team is good enough that there are multiple, realistic options. And add another layer to the bet when your player smacks one out of the park by doubling your bet if he hits another one out during the same game. Double or nothing is always fun.

THE WINNER GETS	....
WHO WON?	....
DATE	....
SPECIAL PROVISIONS	....

LOVE BET #23

For baseball, will there be a squeeze play?

This is when a runner gets caught between two bases, and the other team is trying to tag him out. It's rare, but it does happen. This, too, could be a fun secondary bet.

THE WINNER GETS ....

WHO WON? ....

DATE ....

SPECIAL PROVISIONS ....

LOVE BET #24

What song will be playing in the stadium when you arrive?

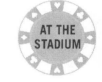

Hint: Familiarize yourself with the most current stadium songs.

THE WINNER GETS ....

WHO WON? ....

DATE ....

SPECIAL PROVISIONS ....

LOVE BET #25

What will the first stadium chant be? ("De-fense!")

It has to be a chant that you hear in the stadium itself, not a chant that you start.

THE WINNER GETS ....

WHO WON? ....

DATE ....

SPECIAL PROVISIONS ....

LOVE BET #26

Will there be a person sitting in your section who has his or her face painted in the team's colors?

Get specific on this one, since this is a Love Bet that causes a lot of controversy. What constitutes "face painted"? The entire face painted or a temporary tattoo on the cheek? And you might want to narrow the area down to three rows in front of your seats and three rows behind. Some stadium sections can have fifty or so rows, so you don't want to have to scan such a huge area for face paint.

THE WINNER GETS	....
WHO WON?	....
DATE	....
SPECIAL PROVISIONS	....

LOVE BET #27

Which team will be the first to score?

This is a 50-50 bet, so it's a safe one to make when this is a first date or when it's early in your relationship. Love Bettors say that the excitement of an impending first score in the game led to a first public kiss, as well as lots of high fives and playful hugs.

THE WINNER GETS	....
WHO WON?	....
DATE	....
SPECIAL PROVISIONS	....

DATE ....

Which type of score will the first one be?

For football, this means a field goal, touchdown, or safety. If one of you isn't too famil-iar with the rules of the game, it's a bonding experience to ask the other to explain.

THE WINNER GETS ....

WHO WON? ....

DATE ....

SPECIAL PROVISIONS ....

Which player will be the first to be booed?

Not just by you, but by the entire crowd? Just be sure that what you hear is, in fact, a boo. It would be embarrassing if you claim (loudly) that you won the bet, and your date has to explain that the crowd is calling out to a player named Bruce or Goose or something similar. Sports fans say they're turned off when their date embarrasses them at the stadium in front of other fans, so don't be attention grabby or argumenta-tive about this bet . . . or any other.

THE WINNER GETS ....

WHO WON? ....

DATE ....

SPECIAL PROVISIONS ....

In football, which end zone will be the site of the first score?

Again, this is a 50-50 bet with you both taking separate end zones and claiming your turf. After the half, you can switch end zones if you'd like.

THE WINNER GETS	....
WHO WON?	....
DATE	....
SPECIAL PROVISIONS	....

Will there be a marriage proposal shown on the scoreboard screen?

This one is a long shot, since it costs a lot of money to get a special message shown on the screen, or to have your proposal filmed out on the field. But it does happen from time to time, so this is one of those slim-odds bets that people make when they get as much happiness from losing the bet as winning, such as in the case of the partner who wants to make a romantic dinner or cash in on a racy wager.

THE WINNER GETS	....
WHO WON?	....
DATE	....
SPECIAL PROVISIONS	....

Will the two of you be featured on kiss cam?

You're just watching the game, and all of a sudden, the screen starts showing pictures of couples in the stands. When you see your image, you're supposed to kiss, and the crowd applauds. If you're on an early date, don't be shy about giving your partner a quick kiss—couples who don't kiss are often booed by the crowd.

THE WINNER GETS	....
WHO WON?	....
DATE	....
SPECIAL PROVISIONS	....

Correctly answer the trivia question shown on the Diamondvision.

During the game, trivia questions are often shown on the big screen. They're usually questions about team or player records and fun stats like "Who was the first player to hit a home run during a full moon on opening day?" Trivia buffs get to show off their smarts, and newcomers to the game can impress their dates with a pretty close guess.

THE WINNER GETS	....
WHO WON?	....
DATE	....
SPECIAL PROVISIONS	....

LOVE BET #34

Will there be a team T-shirt shot into your section?

At minor-league baseball games, stadium staff often run onto the field between innings to catapult team T-shirts into the crowd. Fans consider this giveaway one of the highlights of the game entertainment. You might not be close enough to snag the shirt, but will one be shot into your section? If you really want to up the ante, make a secondary bet that you'll be the one to catch it.

THE WINNER GETS ....

WHO WON? ....

DATE ....

SPECIAL PROVISIONS ....

LOVE BET #35

The first vendor to come to your section will be selling which type of food or drink?

You have your choice of popcorn, hot dogs, beer, cotton candy, peanuts, Cracker Jacks, water, and many other options. This is purely a chance bet and should be made before you reach the stadium. It wouldn't be fair for you to secretly assess the fact that the hot-dog guy is always around and then make the bet.

THE WINNER GETS ....

WHO WON? ....

DATE ....

SPECIAL PROVISIONS ....

LOVE BET #36

How many hot dogs will the person next to you order from the stadium vendor?

Now, be nice about this one, since you don't want your date to think you're judgmental about anyone's eating habits. So go with a low number, since this will surely be a secondary bet among other bets you'll make that day.

THE WINNER GETS ....

WHO WON? ....

DATE ....

SPECIAL PROVISIONS ....

LOVE BET #37

Will the game be called on account of rain, or will the team play through?

If it's a drizzle, the game usually goes on, but if it's a torrential downpour or there's lighting and thunder, they might call the game. So if the weather report says there's a storm brewing, this bet could give you something to do if the game is called early.

THE WINNER GETS ....

WHO WON? ....

DATE ....

SPECIAL PROVISIONS ....

Which kid will win the between-play competition?

At minor league games, kids are often called onto the field between innings to play games and participate in races. You'll both choose a competitor and cheer for them by name as they're announced.

THE WINNER GETS	
WHO WON?	
DATE	
SPECIAL PROVISIONS	

Which team will win the game?

It's best to make this bet at the start of the game, but you can add extra excitement to a close-scoring game or one that goes into extra innings or overtime. The energy in the stadium is up, fans are on their feet, and this is when you can propose your bet.

THE WINNER GETS	
WHO WON?	
DATE	
SPECIAL PROVISIONS	

PART 2
WHAT'S ON TV?

Regardless of what you're watching together, you can add a little wager to your time in front of the tube. If your relationship has sunk into a rut, where watching television is pretty much all you do together, this section can ease your partner into the wager-making mindset. Once your honey sees that a fun bet is on the horizon, you could soon find that he or she is more eager to make bets, and deliver the winnings, in other areas of your life. That's when this book becomes a regular part of your relationship, and that's when things get fun again. So, start with *CSI* or *24* or *American Idol*, or make the red-carpet celebrity-studded awards shows your "thing" for wagering, and see where the romantic wagers take you.

IN THIS EPISODE

PAGE 24

REALITY SHOWS

PAGE 28

AWARDS SHOWS

PAGE 31

LOVE BET #40

Who committed the crime?

You knew it wasn't the obvious suspect the lead characters focused on in the first ten minutes, but a half hour into the show, it could be anybody, the writing is that good. So about twenty minutes into the show, you'll both name your suspects and see who the perp turns out to be.

THE WINNER GETS	....
WHO WON?	....
DATE	....
SPECIAL PROVISIONS	....

LOVE BET #41

What was the evidence that gave it away?

Here's where you get scientific with your knowledge of crime scene science, DNA technology, and criminal psychology. Your date will be impressed when you spot the incriminating evidence or the body language of the lying character.

THE WINNER GETS	....
WHO WON?	....
DATE	....
SPECIAL PROVISIONS	....

LOVE BET #42

Guess the next line the character will say.

Some shows are so cliché and cheesy, it's easy to guess the next piece of dialogue or the character's catchphrase. In *The Office,* for instance, Michael Scott likes to say, "That's what she said" as his comeback to just about any line on the show, so there's a safe bet for you. You'll crack up your date when your lines are better than the characters' lines, so have some fun with this multiple-bets-per-episode choice.

THE WINNER GETS	....
WHO WON?	....
DATE	....
SPECIAL PROVISIONS	....

LOVE BET #43

Solve the cliffhanger from last season.

You'll both have to agree not to look online for spoiler alerts, to keep it fair. Some cliffhangers have completely satisfying resolutions (you never saw it coming) and some are insultingly predictable. Still, this is a great way to share your love of a favorite show and show your creativity and smarts in guessing the outcome.

THE WINNER GETS	....
WHO WON?	....
DATE	....
SPECIAL PROVISIONS	....

LOVE BET #44

When a series regular leaves the show, how will he or she be written off the program?

What happens to the character? Killed off? A transfer to a new hospital? Some programs reveal their plans for a main character, either through promos or on the show website, and others tease you with "A very special episode when (character) says goodbye." Your bet, then, is to guess how that character makes his or her departure. Some Love Bettors like to suggest improbable destinies for characters, such as, "He chucks his law practice to go teach scuba diving in Belize" before settling on their real guess. The first few suggestions can get you laughing together.

THE WINNER GETS	....
WHO WON?	....
DATE	....
SPECIAL PROVISIONS	....

LOVE BET #45

What color will they paint the room?

In just about every home-décor show, they have that moment when the designer pulls out the gallon paint can and pries open the lid with a screwdriver to reveal the color he or she has chosen for the room. In that moment, you both call out your choice of color: "Orange!" "Red!" "Purple!" It's tremendous fun when you guess the most outrageous, unlikely color . . . and you're right!

THE WINNER GETS	....
WHO WON?	....
DATE	....
SPECIAL PROVISIONS	....

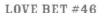

Will they knock out a wall?

Demo is often the best part of home-remodeling shows, whether they use a wrecking ball or a sledge hammer. Some projects require a wall to go and others have the designers knocking out space for a sliding door or window. You choose if there's going to be smashed wallboard or if the place stays intact.

THE WINNER GETS	....
WHO WON?	....
DATE	....
SPECIAL PROVISIONS	....

What will the selling price be?

In most of these shows, they split screen to a budget page, showing what the owner spent to buy the place, how much was invested, and how much he hopes to sell the house for after the redesign. In some episodes, the owner gets more than he wanted, and in some episodes the house hasn't sold and the owner is now living in it. Which will it be for this episode? What's your guess for their profit or loss?

THE WINNER GETS	....
WHO WON?	....
DATE	....
SPECIAL PROVISIONS	....

LOVE BET #48

Which home will they choose?

On some shows, the prospective homebuyers have their choice of House #1, the bungalow by the beach; House #2, the spacious townhouse with the small closets; or House #3, the perfect house right by the freeway. The show gives the pros and cons of each option, then they cut to commercial before they announce which house the buyers chose. That's when you make your bet. If you both agree on the same property, there's no wager this time around. But if you say townhouse and your partner says bungalow, the bet is on!

THE WINNER GETS ....

WHO WON? ....

DATE ....

SPECIAL PROVISIONS ....

LOVE BET #49

Which team will win the challenge?

REALITY
SHOWS

It's not always the youngest team or the team with the brawniest competitors. Some challenges are designed to give the elders the edge, and of course there's always the unforeseen drop of the torch or the mistake that sends them back to the beginning of the obstacle course. You can both root loudly for your team to win.

THE WINNER GETS ....

WHO WON? ....

DATE ....

SPECIAL PROVISIONS ....

LOVE BET #50

What will the reward be?

Since most reality shows reveal the reward before the challenge begins, you should name your guess before the program starts. Will it be soap and toothpaste? A call from home? A helicopter ride with the bachelor or bachelorette? A tray full of waffles and syrup? Toilet paper? Again, this is a bet that allows you to suggest some funny and improbable rewards to show off your sense of humor. Imagine your date's smile when you suggest that island survivors would like a seafood meal when all they've been eating for the past two weeks is fish.

THE WINNER GETS	....
WHO WON?	....
DATE	....
SPECIAL PROVISIONS	....

LOVE BET #51

Which contestants will get romantic during the season?

The show's producers know that we want contestants to hook up, so from the thousands of hours of taped footage, they're likely to show the smooch that two reality show stars share on a drunken night . . . or how they keep warm on that island. To fully enjoy the challenge of this bet, consider making this one when you're watching the first episode of the show and not further into the season when entertainment magazines reveal the budding romance. This way, it's even more fun when your choices of mates turn out to despise each other or fall in love and get engaged on the show's finale.

THE WINNER GETS	....
WHO WON?	....
DATE	....
SPECIAL PROVISIONS	....

LOVE BET #52

Which contestant will eventually be known as "the crazy one"?

There's always a crazy one, and it's not always the one you'd expect. Who's going to alienate everyone on the show and be enough of a drama queen or king to command the most amount of air time during the season? Again, make this bet early in the season and not when the entertainment magazines brand this contestant as the Lunatic or the Ice Queen or the Bad Boy of the show.

THE WINNER GETS	
WHO WON?	
DATE	
SPECIAL PROVISIONS	

LOVE BET #53

Who will get eliminated from the show this week?

As an added level to your wager, you might want to make a secondary bet on if that contestant's "alliance" betrays him or her.

THE WINNER GETS	
WHO WON?	
DATE	
SPECIAL PROVISIONS	

Who will win this season's competition?

You can make this bet at any time during the season, right up until the last show. Bring that contestant's character into your bet, such as making the wager a home-made gumbo if he's Cajun, or a deep-dish pizza if she's from Chicago. If the winner is a sexy, bare-chested carpenter, then perhaps your date can put on a tool belt and play carpenter for you.

THE WINNER GETS	....
WHO WON?	....
DATE	....
SPECIAL PROVISIONS	....

LOVE BET #55

And the winner is . . .

Name the winners in each category, with a mini bet for each one. And theme your wager to the category, such as the gift of a new bra for Best Supporting Actress!

THE WINNER GETS	....
WHO WON?	....
DATE	....
SPECIAL PROVISIONS	....

Predict a political joke made by the show's host, or twist the bet to: Will there be any political jokes in the opening monologue?

These shows are soooo long, that you may not want to watch four hours to catch a political joke made between the award for best sound and the award for best short, so stick to a specific time that the joke will be made, such as within the first half hour or in the last ten minutes.

THE WINNER GETS	
WHO WON?	
DATE	
SPECIAL PROVISIONS	

Who will be named best and worst dressed by your choice of favorite fashion critic?

Granted, it can be hard to get your man to care about fashion, much less bet you on it, but he may be into the worst-dressed category, given some of the really wacky out-fits worn to some of these awards shows. This award is often handed down the day after the awards show, so it's a great secondary bet.

THE WINNER GETS	
WHO WON?	
DATE	
SPECIAL PROVISIONS	

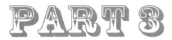
PART 3
WITH FAMILY AND FRIENDS

ake the time you spend with family and friends and add a little twist by wagering on the things that are sure to happen. If you have a bet that Aunt Marge will ask you *again* about when you're going to have a baby, it takes the sting out of the encounter. You won't head right for the desserts; rather, you'll know that you have breakfast in bed coming to you.

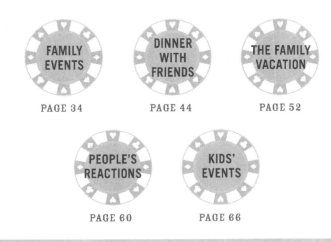

FAMILY EVENTS

PAGE 34

DINNER WITH FRIENDS

PAGE 44

THE FAMILY VACATION

PAGE 52

PEOPLE'S REACTIONS

PAGE 60

KIDS' EVENTS

PAGE 66

At a wedding, what will the happy couple's first-dance song be?

As a secondary bet, will their first dance be choreographed with dips and twirls or will they just dance side to side like at the prom?

THE WINNER GETS	....
WHO WON?	....
DATE	....
SPECIAL PROVISIONS	....

Will there be a line dance at the reception?

We're talking Chicken Dance, The Macarena, The Cha-Cha Slide, you name it. Some couples make it a rule that NO line dances will be performed at their weddings, but someone always gets that request in there. Conga lines count!

THE WINNER GETS	....
WHO WON?	....
DATE	....
SPECIAL PROVISIONS	....

LOVE BET #60

What will the cake topper be?

Mini bride and groom? Monogram letters made of chocolate? Butterflies? Or will the couple go traditional with fresh flowers cascading down the cake?

THE WINNER GETS	....
WHO WON?	....
DATE	....
SPECIAL PROVISIONS	....

LOVE BET #61

Who will be seated at your table?

Will you be with friends, family, strangers, or the kids?

THE WINNER GETS	....
WHO WON?	....
DATE	....
SPECIAL PROVISIONS	....

LOVE BET #62

Will (Guest) bring a date?

There's always that perpetually single cousin or friend, or the relative whose spouse never attends family parties. Will this person show up with an "And Guest"?

THE WINNER GETS	....
WHO WON?	....
DATE	....
SPECIAL PROVISIONS	....

LOVE BET #63

How many times will you be asked when you're getting married?

Or, when you're having a baby, if you're already married. At happy family celebrations, well-meaning relatives always seem to ask The Question. They want the best for you, and they're not trying to be rude. So, you can cut the annoyance factor out of this expected comment by wagering with one another about the number of times you'll hear it!

THE WINNER GETS	....
WHO WON?	....
DATE	....
SPECIAL PROVISIONS	....

LOVE BET #64

Name one cheesy song the deejay or band will play.

In the movie *Love, Actually,* the wedding deejay plays "Puppy Love," which leads the characters to call him the worst deejay ever. Have some fun with the playlist by each choosing a song that would make that deejay the worst ever.

THE WINNER GETS	....
WHO WON?	....
DATE	....
SPECIAL PROVISIONS	....

LOVE BET #65

Will the bride be seen walking around carrying a beer bottle?

The elder generation hates it when brides, dressed in their formal wedding gowns and looking so classy, walk around carrying a bottle of Miller Lite like they're at happy hour. Will the bride at this wedding know enough not to drink out of a bottle?

THE WINNER GETS	....
WHO WON?	....
DATE	....
SPECIAL PROVISIONS	....

LOVE BET #66

Will the bride and groom do the bouquet toss and the garter toss?

In current wedding trends, these two rituals are out of style, and they've become a by-choice element that some wedding couples choose to incorporate into their receptions. Keep in mind that the bride might toss her bouquet, but the groom might not go for the garter—since some families consider that inappropriate with kids at the wedding—so make sure your bet has that provision.

THE WINNER GETS	....
WHO WON?	....
DATE	....
SPECIAL PROVISIONS	....

LOVE BET #67

What will the wedding favor be?

Chocolates? Candy-covered almonds? Little silver frames? Nothing? Some couples are choosing to skip the favors and instead make a donation to charity, so consider that as your possible answer.

THE WINNER GETS	....
WHO WON?	....
DATE	....
SPECIAL PROVISIONS	....

LOVE BET #68

Guess the holiday gifts you will receive, such as gift cards to the bookstore, which you get every year.

If you've dropped hints for a cashmere scarf, will anyone gift you with that elegant present? To better enjoy this bet, each of you can choose three potential gifts that you might receive from other members of the family, not from each other.

THE WINNER GETS	....
WHO WON?	....
DATE	....
SPECIAL PROVISIONS	....

Will your sibling bring a date to the holiday dinner?

If your sister has been dating a nice man for the past six months, will they take the big leap in spending a holiday dinner with your family? Is she up for the scrutiny of that?

THE WINNER GETS	....
WHO WON?	....
DATE	....
SPECIAL PROVISIONS	....

Will anyone announce their engagement during the holiday celebration?

If that brother has been dating a nice girl for several years, is there going to be a big announcement? Will he propose in front of the entire family? When a couple has been together for a long time, many relatives expect an engagement soon, so wager on this holiday being the occasion of joy.

THE WINNER GETS	....
WHO WON?	....
DATE	....
SPECIAL PROVISIONS	....

Will it snow for the holidays?

This bet is especially fun when you live in a region where it could very well snow, but the weather channel is often off-base about *when*, and how much. If you live in an area where it usually does snow, you can tailor your bet to the number of snowfall inches as measured on the news, or with a ruler in your front yard.

THE WINNER GETS	....
WHO WON?	....
DATE	....
SPECIAL PROVISIONS	....

Who will be the first relative to call the family during your holiday celebration?

This could be a happy thing, or one of those eye-rolling moments, such as when your attention-grabbing sister who chose to go skiing in Switzerland instead of spending the holidays with the family calls during the family dinner and wants to talk with everyone about what a great time she's having at the four-star hotel she's staying at. So, either celebrate the good people in your life, or take the edge off the bad, by betting on who's going to make the first phone call.

THE WINNER GETS	....
WHO WON?	....
DATE	....
SPECIAL PROVISIONS	....

LOVE BET #73

Will there be a big argument during the holiday meal?

We don't all have Norman Rockwell families, and the mere mention of a political candidate can start a firestorm of ugly debate, which ends up with someone leaving the table in anger. Happens every time. But you can always hope that it won't. Couples whose families are notorious for dramas during the holidays can turn the awkwardness into a big smile when there's a fun wager attached.

THE WINNER GETS ....

WHO WON? ....

DATE ....

SPECIAL PROVISIONS ....

LOVE BET #74

What will be on the menu?

Every family has traditional dishes that everyone looks forward to enjoying, so which of your family favorites will be on the list?

THE WINNER GETS ....

WHO WON? ....

DATE ....

SPECIAL PROVISIONS ....

What will the theme of the party be?

Fun-loving party hosts can choose really creative themes, especially for family birth-day parties. So think about who's throwing the bash and try to guess what his or her big theme will be this year.

THE WINNER GETS	
WHO WON?	
DATE	
SPECIAL PROVISIONS	

Name a game that will be played at the party.

Some families love board games and others love backyard sports such as badminton and horseshoes. If this is an outdoor summertime party, what's going to be on the game list for the adults or for the kids?

THE WINNER GETS	
WHO WON?	
DATE	
SPECIAL PROVISIONS	

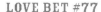

Name a gift that the guest of honor will receive.

It's always fun to guess at the serious or gag gifts that someone will get. Especially for milestone birthdays, the gag gifts are quite predictable (walking canes, Geritol) and the beautiful gifts are breathtaking (pocket watch, an aquamarine birthstone pendant). So decide if you want to go serious or joking with this category before you make your bets.

THE WINNER GETS	....
WHO WON?	....
DATE	....
SPECIAL PROVISIONS	....

Will anyone pull out old family photos?

At family parties and reunions, several generations may be gathered together, so that's the perfect time to share those photo albums and videos from weddings. You can make this bet a general one, such as: Will Grandma pull out the photos? Or you can guess at an All-About-Me cousin who uses the family party to show off her own wedding photos!

THE WINNER GETS	....
WHO WON?	....
DATE	....
SPECIAL PROVISIONS	....

LOVE BET #79

Who will cancel at the last minute, citing babysitter issues?

DINNER
WITH
FRIENDS

We all have those friends, the ones who never follow through on social plans because they can't bear to leave the kids. It becomes an expected thing, so will this be the night that they actually attend a dinner?

THE WINNER GETS	....
WHO WON?	....
DATE	....
SPECIAL PROVISIONS	....

LOVE BET #80

How many times will (Friend) call home to check on the kids?

For new parents, you can expect a lot of calls to be made, sometimes from a cell phone at the dinner table and sometimes during trips to the restroom. Take it easy on these new parents, since it's an understandable thing to have some separation anxiety and worries the first few times out. But when it's a control-freak parent whose kids are older, they're fair game for this bet!

THE WINNER GETS	....
WHO WON?	....
DATE	....
SPECIAL PROVISIONS	....

LOVE BET #81

Will (Friend) talk about his/her newest business venture?

Your friend the entrepreneur is always talking about his new start-up, bragging about his business acumen, and often looking for investors. Will he be in full sales mode tonight?

THE WINNER GETS	....
WHO WON?	....
DATE	....
SPECIAL PROVISIONS	....

LOVE BET #82

Will (Friend) make a reach for the check?

You love your friend, but he's always slow on the draw when it comes to offering to pay for dinner. He makes that halfhearted reach for the check or says, "I was going to pick up the tab" after you've already handed the waiter your credit card. Yeah, sure. Instead of getting aggravated by this person's intrinsic greed, turn him into a bet with a much better outcome.

THE WINNER GETS	....
WHO WON?	....
DATE	....
SPECIAL PROVISIONS	....

LOVE BET #83

How many bottles of wine will you go through as a group?

The last time you went out to dinner with this group of friends, you somehow managed to drink your way through five bottles of wine. Maybe it was a long dinner, service was slow, or there was spillage of a glass or two, but you remember being astounded at the number of bottles on the bill. For this dinner out, will the number of bottles be more or less than those five—or whatever the number was at that last dinner?

THE WINNER GETS	....
WHO WON?	....
DATE	....
SPECIAL PROVISIONS	....

LOVE BET #84

Will your friend tell his or her date what to order for dinner?

It can make you cringe to see a parent-child dynamic of control in a friend's relationship, but if you can't do anything about it, you can share a wager and make the best of it for yourselves.

THE WINNER GETS	....
WHO WON?	....
DATE	....
SPECIAL PROVISIONS	....

Will (Friend) send his dinner back to the kitchen?

In the movie *When Harry Met Sally,* Meg Ryan's character, Sally, was a picky eater. And it was adorable. In the real world, though, it might not be so adorable when a friend is ultra picky about his or her meals and regularly sends a dinner back to the kitchen for a removal of sauce ("I asked for it on the side") or larger broccoli heads or further cooking time. Eyes roll, because it happens every time. Again, instead of getting annoyed by the send back that delays all of your meals, turn it into something fun, a secret bet between the two of you.

THE WINNER GETS	....
WHO WON?	....
DATE	....
SPECIAL PROVISIONS	....

LOVE BET #86

Will (Friend) deliver an emasculating comment to her partner?

She might not order his meal, but she may tell everyone at the table how he's not great at home repairs or how he didn't get a promotion at work. Your bet might include something nice for him, such as delivering a compliment on the paint job he did on their living room, telling him that you love the restaurant he chose—a bit of building up for a friend who could use it. When you're stuck socializing with a friend's horrible spouse or date, you can make it an endeavor to undo the damage. And then treat each other well in your wager, too.

THE WINNER GETS	....
WHO WON?	....
DATE	....
SPECIAL PROVISIONS	....

LOVE BET #87

Will (Friend) gossip about a friend who is not there?

"You know what I heard?" Gossips are insecure, and their idea of fun is ripping apart anyone who's not present to defend themselves. So if you know that a friend or a friend's date is a gossip, you can bet on whether or not he or she will drop a story. If it's a certainty that he or she will gossip, make the bet about whom they tell the tale. Wagers like this make an otherwise unpleasant element of the night something to look forward to, since you get something enjoyable out of it.

THE WINNER GETS	....
WHO WON?	....
DATE	....
SPECIAL PROVISIONS	....

LOVE BET #88

Will (Friend), who is on a diet and talks about it nonstop, order a massive dessert or a fattening meal?

Everyone gets to indulge once in a while, but if this friend is a braggart about how much she works out, how well she diets, or how he just signed on for a boot camp— and, even worse, lectures you about what you're eating—then he or she is fair game as a bet. If the dinner or dessert order is not something Jenny Craig would approve of, one of you wins.

THE WINNER GETS	....
WHO WON?	....
DATE	....
SPECIAL PROVISIONS	....

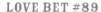

Will the waiter get someone's order wrong?

In a busy restaurant, and especially if you're part of a big group, things can get quite hectic in the kitchen and for your server. So if one of you gets the wrong appetizer or entrée, your bet is on.

THE WINNER GETS	
WHO WON?	
DATE	
SPECIAL PROVISIONS	

Will (Friends) talk endlessly about their latest vacation?

Of course you want to hear about every little thing they did, every meal they ate, the color of every fish they saw while scuba diving, and how many rainbows they saw over the ocean. At least that's what your self-centered friends of friends think, so they try to dominate the conversation with an endless tale of how luxurious their life is. They might even pull out their digital camera to show you photos. If they just returned from their honeymoon, this is understandable, but if it's just another vacation they took then their All-About-Me show could wreck a lovely evening . . . unless you have a Love Bet on it.

THE WINNER GETS	
WHO WON?	
DATE	
SPECIAL PROVISIONS	

LOVE BET #91

Will (Friend) flirt with the waiter?

Especially if she has a few too many glasses of wine in her, one of your friends might be known to get flirty and touchy feely with waiters, bartenders, or the valet. So enjoy her fearlessness by turning her antics into a Love Bet of your own.

THE WINNER GETS	
WHO WON?	
DATE	
SPECIAL PROVISIONS	

LOVE BET #92

Which movie will the group decide to see?

If it hasn't been decided ahead of time, will the vote go toward the action film, the Victorian drama, the romantic comedy, or the animated film? Be fair in letting your date know who will be in attendance so that a better guess can be made.

THE WINNER GETS	
WHO WON?	
DATE	
SPECIAL PROVISIONS	

LOVE BET #93

Will (Friend) take phone calls or return text messages at the table?

This is one of those etiquette don'ts, so it's fair game to make a bet out of rude behavior. Some friends may bring along dates who not only take calls at the table but carry on entire conversations. Again! If this is a known phenomenon in your group of friends, why not turn it into a payoff wager that you can cash in on?

THE WINNER GETS	....
WHO WON?	....
DATE	....
SPECIAL PROVISIONS	....

LOVE BET #94

What time will the evening be done?

This is qualified by the time you walk out of the restaurant or out of your friend's home—not the time you arrive home. If your group of friends regularly stays out until 4:00 A.M., then your bet is about how much stamina you all have that evening. If your friends always seem to make it a one-hour dinner and then a quick hug goodnight, then your bet is: How quickly will the night come to an end?

THE WINNER GETS	....
WHO WON?	....
DATE	....
SPECIAL PROVISIONS	....

LOVE BET #95

At game night, the winner is . . . ?

If you're a couple who enjoys game night—either with friends or on your own—you can make that game of Scrabble, chess, Pictionary, Trivial Pursuit, Scene It, Texas Hold 'Em, or other game the foundation of your own romantic wagers. If you're with a group, extend the practice of fun couple wagers to them as well, and see what they come up with for their own bets. They may just get a relationship jumpstart from your inspiration. If the two of you decide on a racy wager, keep that to yourselves.

THE WINNER GETS	....
WHO WON?	....
DATE	....
SPECIAL PROVISIONS	....

LOVE BET #96

Name the location of this year's family vacation.

THE FAMILY
VACATION

Especially in families where there always seem to be two different camps—with one group wanting a relaxing beach vacation and
the other group wanting to tour European cities or embark on adventure
tours—you'll get to bet on which group's plan will be set. Or, if your family loves the
same style of vacation, which state, city, or island will you all decide on?

THE WINNER GETS	....
WHO WON?	....
DATE	....
SPECIAL PROVISIONS	....

Will your parents expect you to sleep in separate rooms as a matter of respect?

If you've just started dating, or if the parents are really out of touch with reality, your family might require you to sleep in separate rooms. Rather than getting upset about this unfair rule, and thus getting whiny and juvenile, work your way around the rule with a fun Love Bet.

THE WINNER GETS	....
WHO WON?	....
DATE	....
SPECIAL PROVISIONS	....

Who will get the small, crappy room?

You know the room . . . the one with no air conditioning, all the clutter, the room that smells of cigarette smoke, the super-tiny room with the fold-out bed with the bar in the middle of the crappy mattress. Some families play rock-scissors-paper to decide who gets the crappy room, and some families have the martyr sister who takes it and complains the whole week. Who's staying in that room?

THE WINNER GETS	....
WHO WON?	....
DATE	....
SPECIAL PROVISIONS	....

LOVE BET #99

Who will be the first to arrive?

There doesn't have to be a strategy, and you shouldn't bet that you'll be the first ones there, then drive unsafely in a rush. Make this one about the rest of the family. If you're first, who will arrive after you?

THE WINNER GETS	....
WHO WON?	....
DATE	....
SPECIAL PROVISIONS	....

LOVE BET #100

What will be the first restaurant you all go to?

If you're vacationing at the same hotel, shore house, or ski lodge your family traditionally visits, you know the group's favorite places to eat. So, will tonight be the formal restaurant or the barbecue place? The snack bar by the pool? The Irish pub?

THE WINNER GETS	....
WHO WON?	....
DATE	....
SPECIAL PROVISIONS	....

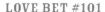

Will (Family Member) attempt the adventure sport offered at the resort?

It might be parasailing, swimming with dolphins, surfing, biking down the side of a volcano. You saw the list on the resort's website, so choose a family member and bet on how adventurous he or she will be during the vacation. Is Mom going to sit out when everyone else goes snorkeling? Is Dad going to offer to take the pictures from the ground while you're up in the parasail?

THE WINNER GETS ....

WHO WON? ....

DATE ....

SPECIAL PROVISIONS ....

Who will try the unique cultural dish or drink?

From poi to tarot root to weird fish dishes and raw meats, who has the brave spirit to sample the local culture?

THE WINNER GETS ....

WHO WON? ....

DATE ....

SPECIAL PROVISIONS ....

LOVE BET #103

What will be the backdrop for the first family photo?

Will it be the beach, a monument, a sign on the highway? The shutterbug of the family will certainly have a styling for the shot, so see if you can guess what the first inspiration will be.

THE WINNER GETS	....
WHO WON?	....
DATE	....
SPECIAL PROVISIONS	....

LOVE BET #104

What will be the activity or game suggested for the first rainy day?

Does the family always do charades? Card games? Will someone suggest that you all watch a movie? Or go shopping? What's the first suggestion going to be?

THE WINNER GETS	....
WHO WON?	....
DATE	....
SPECIAL PROVISIONS	....

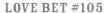

What will your partner forget?

Your partner has forgotten to pack an essential item. It could be a bathing suit, a pair of dress shoes, sun block, and so on.

THE WINNER GETS	....
WHO WON?	....
DATE	....
SPECIAL PROVISIONS	....

Name the first family vacation memory shared by your parents when you ask, "What was the best vacation moment you had with us?"

We all value different memories in different ways, so this bet is a fun way to see if you can guess what your parents hold as the most precious memory. It's often way different from the one you would expect, and when you share *your* guess, you start a great conversation that gives your partner a revealing look into your family history.

THE WINNER GETS	....
WHO WON?	....
DATE	....
SPECIAL PROVISIONS	....

LOVE BET #107

Name a sight you will see on the beach.

Will it be a sunbather in a thong bathing suit, a bodybuilding couple walking along the water's edge, a jogger running with Golden Retriever, a little girl in a too-skimpy bikini for her age? Think about unlikely things as well, for the surprise factor. Will you see someone with a Marilyn Monroe beach towel? Will you see a pink jet ski?

THE WINNER GETS	....
WHO WON?	....
DATE	....
SPECIAL PROVISIONS	....

LOVE BET #108

What will be the first kid's name called out by a nearby parent?

Kids today have great names, so claim your favorite. Will it be Tyler, Caitlin, Isabella, Madison, or another typical kid's name?

THE WINNER GETS	....
WHO WON?	....
DATE	....
SPECIAL PROVISIONS	....

Will you see whales breaching out in the ocean?

At certain times during the year, your location might be on the whale migration path. So you might be able to see pods of whales traveling and the big splash when a whale breaches.

THE WINNER GETS	....
WHO WON?	....
DATE	....
SPECIAL PROVISIONS	....

LOVE BET #110

Will housekeeping leave a mint on your pillow?

Or, if you don't like the mint idea, think about what housekeeping does that's more unique. For instance, on cruises, they might leave towels formed into the shape of an anchor or a puppy with sunglasses on. They often do a different "towel origami" each night, so wager on the shape you'll find when you get back to the room.

THE WINNER GETS	....
WHO WON?	....
DATE	....
SPECIAL PROVISIONS	....

LOVE BET #111

Bet on what souvenirs each other will return with.

Shop separately. Write your bets down and keep them hidden before the shopping spree, to be revealed when you both present your souvenirs.

THE WINNER GETS ....
WHO WON? ....
DATE ....
SPECIAL PROVISIONS ....

LOVE BET #112

Who will be the first to hug you?

If you're from a family of huggers, where you know everyone is going to rush up to you, who will be the first to lift you off the ground?

PEOPLE'S REACTIONS

THE WINNER GETS ....
WHO WON? ....
DATE ....
SPECIAL PROVISIONS ....

LOVE BET #113

Will your mother cry tears of joy?

If you know she's not easily brought to tears it might have to be something really big!

THE WINNER GETS ....
WHO WON? ....
DATE ....
SPECIAL PROVISIONS ....

LOVE BET #114

Who will be the first to say, "I knew it!"

They were onto you. They suspected something was up, even though you did your best to hide the news. Who is the person who can read you so well?

THE WINNER GETS	....
WHO WON?	....
DATE	....
SPECIAL PROVISIONS	....

LOVE BET #115

Name the immature, jealous sibling's reaction: eye roll, leaving the room, making a snide comment like "It's about time!", or changing the subject.

If you have to deal with such a brat, you might as well get something good out of it.

THE WINNER GETS	....
WHO WON?	....
DATE	....
SPECIAL PROVISIONS	....

LOVE BET #116

Who will be the first to offer you advice?

If you've gotten engaged, they'll be the first to tell you who the best caterer is. If you're expecting a baby, they will tell you which vitamins to take. If you closed on a house, they'll suggest their interior decorator. They're loving and helpful, and you adore them for wanting the best for you.

THE WINNER GETS	....
WHO WON?	....
DATE	....
SPECIAL PROVISIONS	....

LOVE BET #117

Will they bring out the champagne and create an impromptu celebration?

If they've been expecting this news for a while, they may have had the champagne chilling. And they prewashed the champagne flutes. If they really knew this was coming, they may have bought a cake or chocolate-dipped strawberries. Is there a cork popping right now?

THE WINNER GETS	....
WHO WON?	....
DATE	....
SPECIAL PROVISIONS	....

LOVE BET #118

Who will propose the first toast to you?

Will it be your parents who lift their glasses to wish you well? A family friend? A grand-parent? Who will think to make this moment extra special?

THE WINNER GETS	....
WHO WON?	....
DATE	....
SPECIAL PROVISIONS	....

LOVE BET #119

Who will say, "Name the baby after me!"

It's something that just about every expecting couple hears from someone. There's always big pressure to "help" name the baby or press for a family namesake. So will it be a pressuring Mom or an adorable niece or nephew whose request is quite innocent?

THE WINNER GETS	....
WHO WON?	....
DATE	....
SPECIAL PROVISIONS	....

LOVE BET #120

Who will be the first person your mother calls on the phone to share the big news?

Will it be her sister? Her best friend? Her therapist? If she doesn't make the call in front of you, ask her who she contacted first.

THE WINNER GETS	....
WHO WON?	....
DATE	....
SPECIAL PROVISIONS	....

LOVE BET #121

Who will be the first to get out the digital camera and video camera?

Cell phone cameras count for this bet, since most people will automatically whip out their cells rather than search for their videocam, unless they knew this big announcement was coming, in which case they have the camera on the tripod awaiting a photo session and family portrait.

THE WINNER GETS	....
WHO WON?	....
DATE	....
SPECIAL PROVISIONS	....

Who will offer to give you a bridal/baby shower or housewarming party?

If you're lucky, it will be tough to decide between several loving, generous friends and relatives who might be the first to offer, which makes this bet all the sweeter.

THE WINNER GETS ....

WHO WON? ....

DATE ....

SPECIAL PROVISIONS ....

If you're pregnant, who will be the first to touch your stomach?

Will anyone try to touch your stomach? This gesture is most often reserved for when you're starting to show, which is when it gets really annoying. So will someone reach out now?

THE WINNER GETS ....

WHO WON? ....

DATE ....

SPECIAL PROVISIONS ....

KIDS' EVENTS

LOVE BET #124

What will the party theme be?

Know that kids' party themes are very creative now, sometimes going beyond the hit kids' cartoon series to a safari theme, beach party in the winter, even science parties where the parents hire zoologists to bring in snakes and turtles for the kids to learn about and hold. It's way different from when we were kids!

THE WINNER GETS	....
WHO WON?	....
DATE	....
SPECIAL PROVISIONS	....

LOVE BET #125

What will be the kids' gaming activity?

Piñata, pony rides, Silly String, a Moonwalk? Again, parents are going way beyond the usual games and investing in marshmallow shooters to simulate paintball, super soakers, petting zoos. How exorbitant are the kiddy games going to be?

THE WINNER GETS	....
WHO WON?	....
DATE	....
SPECIAL PROVISIONS	....

LOVE BET #126

What will be the theme of the birthday cake?

Split your odds by choosing one theme for the party and another for the birthday cake . . . unless you're ultra confident about your choice of theme (such as when a child wants Spiderman every year).

THE WINNER GETS ....

WHO WON? ....

DATE ....

SPECIAL PROVISIONS ....

LOVE BET #127

Name a gift the child will receive.

You may know what the child has been asking for, or the hot toy of the season. One variation on this bet is guessing the title of the video game when it's known that the child is getting the game station or is a big collector.

THE WINNER GETS ....

WHO WON? ....

DATE ....

SPECIAL PROVISIONS ....

Name the slumber-party problem.

When your child is having a slumber party, there's always some sort of mini disaster. Will it be a nosebleed? A broken lamp? A tantrum from homesickness? Vomiting? Will one of the kids wet the bed? Will the kids get into an argument, resulting in your having to call the parent to come get the ousted child? Will the neighbors complain about the noise?

THE WINNER GETS	
WHO WON?	
DATE	
SPECIAL PROVISIONS	

Create a trivia question about your own childhood slumber party, and pose the question to your partner.

For example: True or False? At my slumber party, the boys' soccer team showed up at my window and scared us all with flashlights and howling. We invited them inside for cake and played Spin the Bottle.

THE WINNER GETS	
WHO WON?	
DATE	
SPECIAL PROVISIONS	

Kids' Sporting Events: For the following bets, pick a child in the game that's "your" player. He could be the too-big-for-his-age soccer player or the short-but-quick basketball player. She could be the spitting image of Mia Hamm or the "Eye of the Tiger" kid who's a foot shorter than everyone else on the team. You both choose your player for the day, and all secret, subtle wagering takes place from there. For your own safety, because parents wouldn't appreciate you betting on their kids, create a code such as pulling on your earring or a tap on your partner's leg. And if this is your child you're betting on (or against), you'd better keep it very hush-hush!

LOVE BET #130

Will the player get a hit the first time up at bat?

You'll do this one for each of your players for their first time up at the plate. If your player gets a hit, you win the wager you set before the inning. This is fast-paced play, so have some wagers in mind ahead of time.

THE WINNER GETS	....
WHO WON?	....
DATE	....
SPECIAL PROVISIONS	....

LOVE BET #131

Will the player score?

Will your player be left stranded on base at the end of an inning, or is he or she going to round third and bring it on home? This bet gets very exciting when it's two outs and your player is trying to beat the throw from second base to the catcher. There's a slide and lots of dust, and the umpire takes off his mask to see the action . . . and the runner is . . . safe! Will this mean you win your wager? That kid might be faster than you thought!

THE WINNER GETS	....
WHO WON?	....
DATE	....
SPECIAL PROVISIONS	....

LOVE BET #132

Will there be a home run in the game?

Now keep in mind that in kids' baseball, it's now often considered a home run when the ball drops anywhere in the outfield. No more swinging for the fences. So adjust your wager to take into account the limitations of pint-sized players. You need to know this so that you can adjust your bet accordingly.

THE WINNER GETS	....
WHO WON?	....
DATE	....
SPECIAL PROVISIONS	....

Will the coach yell at your player?

Check the coach out for signs of aggression: a beet-red face, bulging veins, a sloped forehead, pacing, humiliating the seven-year-old players by benching them and then telling off their parents. Cro Magnon coach is in charge. Now make sure you're not being equally offensive by cheering when the coach breaks a kid's spirit or uses inappropriate language. This bet is simply predicting if the coach is going to say, "You should have thrown it to first base," not "Someone should slap your mother for how bad a player you are." If the coach is truly heinous, then cancel the bet and make a call to the school or town recreation center to report this awful coach's behavior.

THE WINNER GETS ....

WHO WON? ....

DATE ....

SPECIAL PROVISIONS ....

Will any parent lose control and start screaming obscenities at the coach, ref, or umpire?

Now we have Cro Magnon parent, someone who's had too many Red Bulls, is aggressive and combative, insulting, bullying, and socially unacceptable. While all you can do with a nitwit parent when the kid's not in danger is shake your head, why not place a little wager on whether some parent will flip their lid and take their "living vicariously" frustrations out on the coach.

THE WINNER GETS ....

WHO WON? ....

DATE ....

SPECIAL PROVISIONS ....

LOVE BET #135

Can you guess my greatest childhood sports accomplishment?

Rather than leave it wide open, give your partner four options: When I was a kid, I was: A). The winning runner in the state semi-finals game; B). The player all the coaches wanted to draft, and the coaches would fight over it; C). Voted team captain because of my motivational skills; D). The record holder for the most sit-ups in sixty seconds during state physical fitness testing, and my record still stands. This bet is way more fun when you show off your creativity and sense of humor, and when you make it just hard enough.

THE WINNER GETS	....
WHO WON?	....
DATE	....
SPECIAL PROVISIONS	....

LOVE BET #136

Which team will win the game?

If it's a close one, this is a fun bet. If it's a blowout, you can adjust your bet to a point spread such as: Will the team win by less than fifteen points or runs?

THE WINNER GETS	....
WHO WON?	....
DATE	....
SPECIAL PROVISIONS	....

By how many points?

You can do a points spread for any game, whether it's a close call or a blowout. You can turn this bet into a double-or-nothing by betting on who wins and by how much to bring the stakes up a little higher. Instead of just a hot dog at the concessions stand for the one who guessed the win, make it a full barbecue meal at home if you guess the winner and the point spread.

THE WINNER GETS	....
WHO WON?	....
DATE	....
SPECIAL PROVISIONS	....

Will the star player be hoisted up and carried off the field?

It might be a grand slam, a home run, or a throw that turns a double play to end the game . . . or win the championship. When the player saves the day, his or her team-mates will often enact an age-old tradition of carrying the hero off the field. Will you see that victorious ride today?

THE WINNER GETS	....
WHO WON?	....
DATE	....
SPECIAL PROVISIONS	....

Where is the team heading for a post-game celebration?

An ice cream place? A pizza place? The coach's house for a swim party? Or does everyone just go home and do homework? Find out if and how things have changed for kids on sports teams.

THE WINNER GETS	....
WHO WON?	....
DATE	....
SPECIAL PROVISIONS	....

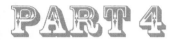

PART 4
COUPLE'S
ALONE TIME

These bets are for your alone time on date nights out on the town or on a vacation that you take as a couple. You may have a lot on your vacation agenda, but there's always time for a little friendly betting.

ON THE TOWN

PAGE 76

ON VACATION

PAGE 83

How many minutes will you have to wait for a table?

ON THE TOWN

Forget what time your reservation was for. Some of the most posh, chic eateries in the city consider it an honor for you to wait an hour for your table to be ready, so rather than get steamed as you order a $20 cocktail at the bar, turn this wait into a wager. Draw four circles on a cocktail napkin, each one representing a fifteen-minute wait. You each put your name in two circles. When you're called for your table, the winner's name is in the circle of that timing. What's your strategy? Take the first two circles? The last two? Mix it up?

THE WINNER GETS	
WHO WON?	
DATE	
SPECIAL PROVISIONS	

LOVE BET #141

Pick out one person sitting at the bar or at a table. What will that person order for his or her drink?

A premium beer or a microbrew? A fruity cocktail or a stiff drink? You can never tell by looking at a person what their drink will be, and people watching is a prime bonding experience, especially on a first or early date. Guess The Drink is one of the top choices for Love Bets.

THE WINNER GETS	
WHO WON?	
DATE	
SPECIAL PROVISIONS	

What will that person order for his or her meal?

Buffalo wings for an after-work snack? A healthy salad with a whole-wheat roll? A drippy, messy pizza burger with fries? What will be the topping on that group's pizza? Is that a pepperoni crowd or a veggie-topping crowd? Again, you can't tell from looking at people how they will order, so it's fun to see if your nonscientific guess has the odds in your favor.

THE WINNER GETS ....

WHO WON? ....

DATE ....

SPECIAL PROVISIONS ....

Will your waiter be male or female?

Especially on early-in-the-relationship dates, this one is fun to choose, since it's a safe 50-50 bet. And the waiter will wonder why you're so happy to see him or her.

THE WINNER GETS ....

WHO WON? ....

DATE ....

SPECIAL PROVISIONS ....

Name a song that the pianist or entertainment will perform.

This one is fun, no matter how long you've been together. The finger-snappin', head boppin' Sinatra-wannabe singer is sure to sing "The Lady is a Tramp," or a very dramatic "My Way." You'll both choose your expected songs, and the winner is the one whose song is performed first.

THE WINNER GETS	
WHO WON?	
DATE	
SPECIAL PROVISIONS	

Will the waiter present the check to one of you or place it in the middle of the table?

At the end of the meal, the waiter will approach the table carrying that little leather folder containing your check. Even if one of you took the initiative to wave down the waiter to signify you're ready to pay, that waiter can make an in-the-moment decision of who will get that folder. Some waiters, very amusingly, *guess* at who will foot the bill, such as handing it to the guy in the suit, or the woman at the head of the table. Some just drop it in the middle of the table and let guests decide how to handle it.

THE WINNER GETS	
WHO WON?	
DATE	
SPECIAL PROVISIONS	

Will you get access to the VIP area?

It's no reflection on how hot you look—cranky gatekeepers have been known to keep the velvet rope closed for all but the A-list. Will this be your lucky night, and will you gain entry into the elite lounge?

THE WINNER GETS	....
WHO WON?	....
DATE	....
SPECIAL PROVISIONS	....

LOVE BET #147

Name a song that will be played in the club.

What are the usual songs that are hot right now? What's the trendiest new release? If you're at a theme bar, such as an '80s club, name a song that will be on the playlist, such as anything from *The Breakfast Club* or Duran Duran. If you're both club goers, you know which songs are going to be played; all that matters to you now is which one will be heard first.

THE WINNER GETS	....
WHO WON?	....
DATE	....
SPECIAL PROVISIONS	....

Will there be a woman with a silver halter top?

At the time of this writing, the silver halter top was the in choice. What will it be today? Choose your own stereotypical club outfit according to what you've seen in the fashion and entertainment magazines, or what the celebutantes have been captured wearing by the paparazzi.

THE WINNER GETS	....
WHO WON?	....
DATE	....
SPECIAL PROVISIONS	....

Will there be a limousine parked outside the nightclub?

It doesn't have to be a celebrity's limo; bachelorette parties travel by stretch limo all the time, as do couples who have just gotten engaged, groups of friends on a big celebratory night out, and, of course, the D-list celebrity who wants to be noticed.

THE WINNER GETS	....
WHO WON?	....
DATE	....
SPECIAL PROVISIONS	....

LOVE BET #150

Will you run into friends while out at the club?

If you were lucky enough to get in, will they also make it inside? Will you see them outside, waiting in line to get in? Are these friends who aren't supposed to be at any nightclub, whether due to their age or their promise to stop clubbing? You can twist this bet any way you'd like.

> **THE WINNER GETS** ....
> **WHO WON?** ....
> **DATE** ....
> **SPECIAL PROVISIONS** ....

LOVE BET #151

While inside the club, will your friend successfully ask someone to dance with him/her?

If you've gone in a group with other friends, a single among you might find the courage to ask someone to dance. Will he lead his target to the dance floor or will he crash and burn? If you watched "The Pickup Artist" on television, you know how much fun it can be to observe singles on the prowl. So, wager up and see if that first target will say yes or no, and get ready to double the wager for the single's next approach.

> **THE WINNER GETS** ....
> **WHO WON?** ....
> **DATE** ....
> **SPECIAL PROVISIONS** ....

LOVE BET #152

How many phone calls will you have missed during your night out?

Of course, you've been polite and turned your cell off while out on a date! If your date knows that you get a lot of calls for work, or even if your date doesn't know that every friend you have has offered to make the "rescue call" in case the date goes badly, that missed-call count can be pretty high. Be careful with this one on a first date or on early dates, since a high call count could give the impression that you're dating other people . . . and they all called you tonight.

THE WINNER GETS	....
WHO WON?	....
DATE	....
SPECIAL PROVISIONS	....

LOVE BET #153

If you've left the kids with a babysitter, what will the babysitter be doing when you get home?

Watching TV? Talking on the phone? Texting? Turning off your computer as fast as possible? Doing homework? Standing in the doorway looking really guilty?

THE WINNER GETS	....
WHO WON?	....
DATE	....
SPECIAL PROVISIONS	....

Will your flight depart on time?

With all of the travel trouble going on at airports, it's almost a rarity
when flights *are* on time. Optimists will bet "Yes" and pessimists will
likely take the "No way!" stance. This bet is best made the day before
the flight, making sure no one can cheat by checking flight status online on the way
to the airport or getting flight delay text messages from the airline on the day of travel.

ON VACATION

THE WINNER GETS	....
WHO WON?	....
DATE	....
SPECIAL PROVISIONS	....

If not, how long will the flight be delayed?

Make separate bets for each block of time: under half an hour; between half an hour
and an hour; one to two hours; more than two hours. Stick with just those four categories, since you don't want to annoy everyone around you in the airport by calling
out for a time check too often. Guessing times for delayed departures—whether it's
for a train, cruise, flight, or cab ride—takes the sting out of waiting and can even get
you laughing when time drags on and on.

THE WINNER GETS	....
WHO WON?	....
DATE	....
SPECIAL PROVISIONS	....

LOVE BET #156

Will there be a crying baby on the plane?

Not a cooing, gurgling baby. Not baby noises. A crying baby. And double the bet if there is more than one crying baby on the flight—it's a great secondary bet.

THE WINNER GETS	....
WHO WON?	....
DATE	....
SPECIAL PROVISIONS	....

LOVE BET #157

Name the in-flight movie choice.

Some airlines will give you a choice of several feature films, usually movies that have just appeared in the theaters, so think about what was just playing at the multiplex. Agree that neither of you will call the airline or check online to find this out!

THE WINNER GETS	....
WHO WON?	....
DATE	....
SPECIAL PROVISIONS	....

Will you have a chatty pilot who turns your flight into an educational program, mentioning landmarks out the windows, sharing FYIs about where you're headed, etc.?

In order to make your flight memorable, or endear you to an airline that's competing with other carriers for your business, some pilots consider it a fun customer service perk to give you a guided tour of what you're flying past. Some pilots make jokes, and others will just provide the facts such as arrival time and the weather at your destination. Which type of pilot are you going to get?

THE WINNER GETS	
WHO WON?	
DATE	
SPECIAL PROVISIONS	

LOVE BET #159

How many times will you circle in a holding pattern before landing at your destination?

This one is only possible if you're low enough to spot a landmark and track how many times you're circling.

THE WINNER GETS	
WHO WON?	
DATE	
SPECIAL PROVISIONS	

LOVE BET #160

Each of you choose a song that will play next on the radio.

For top forty stations, you know the chart toppers they play over and over and over again, so take your pick. If you'd like more of a challenge, select a radio station you've never listened to before, such as easy jazz or retro hits, alternative music or a college radio station, and then try to guess the next song. This bet offers quite a scale from easy to difficult, and it can make a long car ride a veritable fountain of fun wagers.

THE WINNER GETS	
WHO WON?	
DATE	
SPECIAL PROVISIONS	

LOVE BET #161

What will be the company name on the next truck you see?

FedEx? Poland Spring? If you're on a stretch of highway in a faraway region and you're noticing a lot of local trucks rather than trailers from chain stores, guess the category of company name, such as an exterminator or a furniture store.

THE WINNER GETS	
WHO WON?	
DATE	
SPECIAL PROVISIONS	

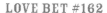

LOVE BET #162

Choose a type of car, from hybrid coupe to SUV, Lexus to VW Bug. Now bet on the color of the next one you see.

Betting on a car type is way too easy, so ramp up the challenge by giving this one a color variable. Or, if you're not up on your car makes and models, you'll each choose an unusual color (like purple or mint green) and look for the first vehicle in that color on the road.

THE WINNER GETS ....

WHO WON? ....

DATE ....

SPECIAL PROVISIONS ....

LOVE BET #163

Play spot the speed trap and guess where the police car will be hiding, such as behind the next overpass, over that hill, in a side street, and so on.

Just make sure you're driving the speed limit while you're sharing this bet, since you don't want to start any explanation about the bet with, "What seems to be the problem, Officer?"

THE WINNER GETS ....

WHO WON? ....

DATE ....

SPECIAL PROVISIONS ....

Will you get the view you asked for at the hotel?

Sure, you may have gotten a terrific rate through your travel discount club, by using your frequent flier mileage, or by booking a special at the travel agent, but did you really get that beachfront bungalow? Is your room fully ocean view, or do you have to open the window and lean way out to even see the ocean? Creating a wager for this portion of your getaway removes a great deal of aggravation about not getting the room of your dreams. If you win, you may get something much better.

THE WINNER GETS	....
WHO WON?	....
DATE	....
SPECIAL PROVISIONS	....

Guess the floor your room will be on.

Even if you specifically asked for first floor, you never know where the booking agent will assign you.

THE WINNER GETS	....
WHO WON?	....
DATE	....
SPECIAL PROVISIONS	....

Will there be a wedding at your hotel that weekend?

You can ask when you check in, but be aware that some hotel chains will not give out that kind of information to protect the privacy of the wedding couple. Yes, you'll see the guests milling about and the bride posing for photos, but the front desk might not tell you if there's a wedding planned, for fear that you're planning to crash the party. It's far better to make this bet before you check in, and look for wedding signs or bridal-party members that evening.

THE WINNER GETS	....
WHO WON?	....
DATE	....
SPECIAL PROVISIONS	....

Name the convention that will be taking place at your hotel.

Dentists? Lawyers? Comic-book geeks? Pharmaceutical reps? Right now, there are a lot of wedding-industry conventions going on, with lots of hotel chains inviting wedding coordinators to visit due to the rising popularity of destination weddings, so that might be a category to consider for your bet.

THE WINNER GETS	....
WHO WON?	....
DATE	....
SPECIAL PROVISIONS	....

Will you hear the next-door room occupants through the wall?

Notice we haven't specified what you can hear, so any noise counts, not just the sounds of intimacy. It could be the television set, children at play, loud talking on the phone, the hair dryer—any noise that's coming from the next room and not the hallway counts.

THE WINNER GETS	....
WHO WON?	....
DATE	....
SPECIAL PROVISIONS	....

Guess the price of a mini-bar item.

Is that pack of M&Ms over or under $3, for instance? What about the tiny bottle of vodka? Over or under $8? Be very careful to read the rules of the mini bar before you play this one, since some mini bars use a sensor that will charge you if you remove an item from the mini bar for more than ten seconds. So don't pull everything out of the mini bar for this bet, or you'll get slapped with a huge bill, even if you put everything back and didn't eat or drink a thing!

THE WINNER GETS	....
WHO WON?	....
DATE	....
SPECIAL PROVISIONS	....

LOVE BET #170

What will be the color of the specialty frozen drink?

When you're staying at an all-inclusive hotel where the $15 frozen margaritas are already paid for in the price of your stay, you'll notice that the daily special is some shade of neon. So which color will it be today? Bright pink? Bright blue? Piña-colada white? This can turn into a daily wager.

THE WINNER GETS	....
WHO WON?	....
DATE	....
SPECIAL PROVISIONS	....

LOVE BET #171

Guess which kind of dive the person on the diving board will do.

The first time you make this bet, you're going to vastly underestimate the small child who's standing in line for the diving board. No, the kid isn't learning to dive. he or she can probably do a triple tuck with a twist. For adult divers, will it be head first or feet first? A cannonball or jackknife?

THE WINNER GETS	....
WHO WON?	....
DATE	....
SPECIAL PROVISIONS	....

LOVE BET #172

Pick the first surfer to fall off his or her board.

Will it be the one in the red surf shorts, the yellow bikini, the black wetsuit with the yellow stripes? The showoff? You don't want anyone to get hurt, of course; you're just looking for regular wipeouts.

THE WINNER GETS	....
WHO WON?	....
DATE	....
SPECIAL PROVISIONS	....

LOVE BET #173

How many girls will be standing around the lifeguard stand?

It's Flirtation Central as a half-dozen girls in bikinis compete for the attention of the bronzed-god lifeguards, and there's lots of hair flipping going on as the fun-to-watch pickup scene unfolds right there in front of you. Were you ever one of those girls, trying to get the lifeguards' attention during summers at the beach? Were you ever the lifeguard in demand? As a fun side story to this bet, share the tale with your partner now.

THE WINNER GETS	....
WHO WON?	....
DATE	....
SPECIAL PROVISIONS	....

Name an item we'll see lying at the edge of the ocean.

It could be a jellyfish, a clamshell, a piece of blue sea glass, a child's abandoned toy—you name it. This bet introduced the option of taking a hand-in-hand stroll along the water's edge. As you search for bet items, you're getting a romantic walk together.

THE WINNER GETS	....
WHO WON?	....
DATE	....
SPECIAL PROVISIONS	....

Will there be a dolphin sighting out in the ocean?

It might be a single dolphin or it might be a whole group of them, in one of the most beautiful sights possible on any beach.

THE WINNER GETS	....
WHO WON?	....
DATE	....
SPECIAL PROVISIONS	....

LOVE BET #176

Will any other vacationers invite you to join them for a meal or activity?

If you're the gregarious types, you might strike up a conversation with the family next to you at dinner or at the pool, and you have insta-friends during the trip. Some lifetime friendships have started this way, with e-mail keeping them close and future vacations planned together. At some shore towns where everyone rents a beach house for the same week in the summer, new communities form where it's the same people around you each year.

THE WINNER GETS	....
WHO WON?	....
DATE	....
SPECIAL PROVISIONS	....

LOVE BET #177

Will you see an eel while snorkeling or scuba diving?

Choose your own type of sea life for this one: sea turtle, stingray, and so on. Before you take your orientation classes and set out for your dive, agree on the type of sea life you'll each claim for your bet.

THE WINNER GETS	....
WHO WON?	....
DATE	....
SPECIAL PROVISIONS	....

LOVE BET #178

How many people will ask if you're on your honeymoon?

If you're really acting like you're in love, you can bet that many people will ask. It seems everyone wants to "catch" some of the romance you're displaying, so don't be afraid to hold hands, kiss, hug, dance close during a slow song, and so on.

THE WINNER GETS	
WHO WON?	
DATE	
SPECIAL PROVISIONS	

LOVE BET #179

The first foreign language you will hear spoken will be _____.

Will it be melodic French or unmistakable Chinese? Or, you might decide to go with an accent rather than a foreign language, since some of the Slavic languages can be difficult to tell apart. You might have more fun betting on overhearing southern accents or a Boston twang.

THE WINNER GETS	
WHO WON?	
DATE	
SPECIAL PROVISIONS	

LOVE BET #180

Will the hot tub be too crowded to get in?

If the hot tub is the big draw due to its beautiful setting and view of the ocean, you might find there's no room during the afternoon hours—everyone is there when you first check it out. Your bet, then, is whether or not your first attempt will be successful.

THE WINNER GETS	....
WHO WON?	....
DATE	....
SPECIAL PROVISIONS	....

LOVE BET #181

Will you interrupt a couple who was getting intimate in the hot tub?

They won't make eye contact with you, and there's a lot of bathing suit adjusting going on. You might decide to walk away and leave them alone, or you might decide to hop in.

THE WINNER GETS	....
WHO WON?	....
DATE	....
SPECIAL PROVISIONS	....

How many times will your ski instructor use the word "dude"?

Choose any ski slang you'd like, such as "bra" or "gnarly." The more stereotypical the better, since many vacationers attempt to fit in by talking like snowboarders do.

THE WINNER GETS	....
WHO WON?	....
DATE	....
SPECIAL PROVISIONS	....

Will you see a celebrity at the ski lodge?

Some winter ski resorts are havens for celebrities, especially if there's a big event taking place nearby, such as film festivals or ski competitions. So make this bet a yes or no answer, since it would be too hard to try to guess which celebrity you'll see. Enjoy the banter when you see a D-lister and debate over whether or not he or she counts as a celebrity.

THE WINNER GETS	....
WHO WON?	....
DATE	....
SPECIAL PROVISIONS	....

LOVE BET #184

How low will the temperature get?

Check the weather report first thing in the morning to see how low the temperature got overnight. Did you hit negative numbers? Whoever's guess is closest wins.

THE WINNER GETS ....

WHO WON? ....

DATE ....

SPECIAL PROVISIONS ....

LOVE BET #185

Will your flight home be on time?

Again, use those half-hour increments to multiply your wagering fun.

THE WINNER GETS ....

WHO WON? ....

DATE ....

SPECIAL PROVISIONS ....

LOVE BET #186

What will await you when you return home?

For example, the house sitter has had a party and things got broken, a package will be waiting by your front door, you'll have over twenty voice mails, and so on.

THE WINNER GETS ....

WHO WON? ....

DATE ....

SPECIAL PROVISIONS ....

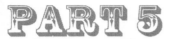

PART 5
WORK EVENTS

I t could be your work conference or office holiday party, or your partner's, and one of you may not exactly be thrilled about going to yet another obligatory social function with colleagues and bosses. The small talk, the cocktails, the inter-office politics thinly veiled by planned festivities. This is often a necessary attendance function, but one that's very important to your or your partner's career. So rather than tough it out or swallow down glass after glass of Pinot just waiting for it to be over, make an event of it with a romantic wager or two. No one from the office needs to know; it'll be your little secret.

OFFICE OUTINGS

PAGE 100

THE HOLIDAY PARTY

PAGE 102

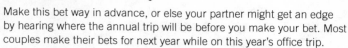

LOVE BET #187

Where will the office conference destination be this year?

OFFICE OUTINGS

Make this bet way in advance, or else your partner might get an edge by hearing where the annual trip will be before you make your bet. Most couples make their bets for next year while on this year's office trip.

THE WINNER GETS	....
WHO WON?	....
DATE	....
SPECIAL PROVISIONS	....

LOVE BET #188

Will you get an ocean-view room or a view of the parking lot?

Employees probably won't get the best rooms in the resort, so have some fun with the collection of bad-view or small-bed rooms. You won't spend too much time in them, with all of those group activities planned, so use them more for fun and romantic wagers.

THE WINNER GETS	....
WHO WON?	....
DATE	....
SPECIAL PROVISIONS	....

LOVE BET #189

Name one of the activities planned on the itinerary.

Will there be a company luau? An obstacle course? A winery tour? A sports tournament with each department competing with the others? Hopefully, your company doesn't do the same old thing each year and there are plenty of odds for variety.

THE WINNER GETS ....

WHO WON? ....

DATE ....

SPECIAL PROVISIONS ....

LOVE BET #190

For any sporting competition, which team will win?

Will you join the cheering section for corporate or will you cheer for the IT staff? Obviously, it could be bad for your position in the company if you're trash talking the boss, so this could be a bet you'll keep just between the two of you.

THE WINNER GETS ....

WHO WON? ....

DATE ....

SPECIAL PROVISIONS ....

LOVE BET #191

Which colleague will bring along the rent-a-date?

Take your pick from the single men and women in your office—those not in a serious relationship—and see who will bring a date to the event, rather than attend alone. Did they find this person on the Internet? Is this a very awkward second date? Does your colleague pay appropriate attention to the date or is he off with the guys, leaving the date with the wives?

THE WINNER GETS	....
WHO WON?	....
DATE	....
SPECIAL PROVISIONS	....

LOVE BET #192

Will (Colleague) be all over his or her date?

THE HOLIDAY PARTY

There's nothing like an open bar to bring out the PDAs; so is your chosen colleague making out in the corner with the date, dancing way too suggestively, disappearing into the coat closet for some action?

THE WINNER GETS	....
WHO WON?	....
DATE	....
SPECIAL PROVISIONS	....

Will (Colleague's) antisocial spouse attend?

He never comes to these things. He's working at home. He's home sick. He couldn't care less about her job or her work life. Whatever the excuse, the guy never comes to office events and parties. So will this be the year that he puts on the Rudolph light-up tie and joins the festivities?

THE WINNER GETS	....
WHO WON?	....
DATE	....
SPECIAL PROVISIONS	....

Will the boss wear a holiday-themed item of clothing?

A red shirt doesn't count. We're talking a sweater with Rudolph on it or a tie with light-up Christmas ornaments, or dreidel-shaped earrings, or a snowman pin. There has to be a holiday icon on it.

THE WINNER GETS	....
WHO WON?	....
DATE	....
SPECIAL PROVISIONS	....

LOVE BET #195

Name an item of food on the menu.

Will there be mini crab cakes? Shrimp cocktail? Pigs in blankets? A cheese plate? Does your office party planner always get the same catering choices, or is your office known for its unique and exciting menus?

THE WINNER GETS	....
WHO WON?	....
DATE	....
SPECIAL PROVISIONS	....

LOVE BET #196

Who will walk around with the sprig of mistletoe, looking for a kiss?

There's always "that guy" who thinks it's funny. Even better, there's always "that guy" who walks around with a sprig of rosemary stolen off the turkey, calling it mistletoe and looking for a kiss.

THE WINNER GETS	....
WHO WON?	....
DATE	....
SPECIAL PROVISIONS	....

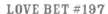

Will any colleague be seen fastening the mistletoe to his belt buckle?

Yes, there's always "that guy" who thinks that's funny.

THE WINNER GETS	
WHO WON?	
DATE	
SPECIAL PROVISIONS	

Name one cheesy holiday song that will be played at the party.

And by "cheesy," we're talking gimmicky, not a holiday classic. It's "Grandma Got Run Over By a Reindeer," not Bing Crosby's "White Christmas."

THE WINNER GETS	
WHO WON?	
DATE	
SPECIAL PROVISIONS	

LOVE BET #199

Will you know everyone's name in order to introduce your date?

Oooo, the pressure! Will you remember your colleagues' spouses' names? Will you go blank? This is a challenging bet—thankfully, in play only at the start of the party.

THE WINNER GETS	....
WHO WON?	....
DATE	....
SPECIAL PROVISIONS	....

LOVE BET #200

Will the holiday décor include a singing or musical plush toy?

From singing penguins to Christmas Yoda, the catalogs are full of interactive holiday toys. So either make this one a yes or no bet or up the ante by claiming that the winner has to name the dancing plush toy.

THE WINNER GETS	....
WHO WON?	....
DATE	....
SPECIAL PROVISIONS	....

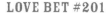

Will (Colleague) get drunk and hit on another colleague?

Everyone knows that Jill in accounting has had the hots for Jim in legal, and every-one knows that Jill can't hold her liquor. So will she gain some liquid courage and make a play for him? Play fair; don't buy drinks for Jill and don't facilitate the hookup by sending them both to the bar at the same time. This has to be a natural approach.

THE WINNER GETS ....
WHO WON? ....
DATE ....
SPECIAL PROVISIONS ....

Will (Colleague) be unable to snap out of work mode, spending the whole night still talking about business?

Frank's always closing. He's obsessed with his new project or freaking out about his new client. The guy doesn't know how to switch into social mode, so will this be the night he just relaxes and has fun?

THE WINNER GETS ....
WHO WON? ....
DATE ....
SPECIAL PROVISIONS ....

LOVE BET #203

Will (Flirty Colleague) wear a low-cut, revealing blouse?

Before you nominate her for "What Not To Wear" for a new, office-appropriate wardrobe, create a yes-no wager on her choice of attire for the party.

THE WINNER GETS	
WHO WON?	
DATE	
SPECIAL PROVISIONS	

LOVE BET #204

Will there be a big announcement at the party, such as the location of the next company vacation, the top salesperson for the year, raises for everyone, a new partner named, and so on?

With everyone gathered in one place, the bosses may decide that it would be great for team morale to publicly recognize the top performers in the company—which is often suggested in articles on boosting team productivity. Bosses also like to spring good company news on the staff during a time when everyone's more relaxed, and also when spouses are in the room. Bosses know that spouses often hear the dark side of working for the company, so they may choose to look like a hero by taking this time to share positive news.

THE WINNER GETS	
WHO WON?	
DATE	
SPECIAL PROVISIONS	

PART 6
MIX IT UP

The things in your everyday life—not just while you're on dates or vacations—are perfect for spicing up your wagers. So this might be the section you come to most often for those fun little bets that make a plain Tuesday night an opportunity to share a playful moment.

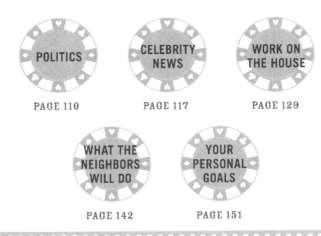

POLITICS

PAGE 110

CELEBRITY NEWS

PAGE 117

WORK ON THE HOUSE

PAGE 129

WHAT THE NEIGHBORS WILL DO

PAGE 142

YOUR PERSONAL GOALS

PAGE 151

Who will be your party's chosen presidential and vice presidential candidates?

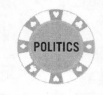

POLITICS

Make this one way in advance, since political coverage extends for over a year, and it's often not a surprise at all who wins the nomination.

THE WINNER GETS	
WHO WON?	
DATE	
SPECIAL PROVISIONS	

What will their theme song be?

Politicians love to mix in a little bit of popular culture, so which song are they going to claim as their "running soundtrack." Which song will be playing as the balloons drop?

THE WINNER GETS	
WHO WON?	
DATE	
SPECIAL PROVISIONS	

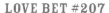

Name the next celebrity to step in front of the camera to endorse the candidates.

You know which celebrities are most outspoken about politics, and you may even have heard the list of stars slated to appear at the convention. But which celebrity will be the first to be shown on air? If you've chosen a celebrity couple, such as Susan Sarandon and Tim Robbins, and they walk out on stage together, it's either a draw or you could slow motion your DVR to see which celebrity stepped onto the stage first.

THE WINNER GETS ....
WHO WON? ....
DATE ....
SPECIAL PROVISIONS ....

LOVE BET #208

Name the next photo op you see together.

Will your candidate serve food at a soup kitchen, visit injured veterans, kiss that baby, visit the troops, dance with a salsa troupe? Politicians love to show their dedication to certain causes, and the nightly news does love to show them in action, so what's the scene going to be the next time the two of you are watching television together? Again, the bet is only valid when you're both together. No e-mailed YouTube footage allowed.

THE WINNER GETS ....
WHO WON? ....
DATE ....
SPECIAL PROVISIONS ....

LOVE BET #209

What will be the destination of the sitting president's next overseas trip?

If the president is known for taking a lot of trips, you have a world of options open to you. Will it be Greece? India? The Sudan? Make sure this isn't a summit that's been publicized for months; choose the unexpected excursion.

THE WINNER GETS ....

WHO WON? ....

DATE ....

SPECIAL PROVISIONS ....

LOVE BET #210

What will be the next big political scandal?

Drug use? Cheating? Illegal nanny? A leaked voice mail in which a senator insults every socio-political group? Our leaders can show some pretty questionable behavior sometimes, so what's going to be the next firestorm?

THE WINNER GETS ....

WHO WON? ....

DATE ....

SPECIAL PROVISIONS ....

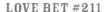

LOVE BET #211

Who will be the next head of state to visit the White House?

If you share a love of politics, this bet will be right up your alley. Plus, you can show off your smarts by being able to name the various presidents and prime ministers of various countries.

THE WINNER GETS	....
WHO WON?	....
DATE	....
SPECIAL PROVISIONS	....

LOVE BET #212

Will the Supreme Court Justice candidate be approved?

Whenever a president nominates a possible Supreme Court Justice, politicians go wild to either support or condemn that candidate. The nomination hearings can be quite dramatic, so if you follow the proceedings together, you can wager on the outcome.

THE WINNER GETS	....
WHO WON?	....
DATE	....
SPECIAL PROVISIONS	....

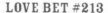

LOVE BET #213

Will there be a unanimous vote on the big issue in Congress?

The issue in question can seem like a no-brainer, such as extra money for disaster relief or funds for cancer research—whatever bill is on the table.

THE WINNER GETS ....

WHO WON? ....

DATE ....

SPECIAL PROVISIONS ....

LOVE BET #214

Who will be the first candidate to drop out of the race in the early months?

A year or so before a big election—sometimes even earlier—the enormous field of candidates gets winnowed down. In gubernatorial elections especially, you'll always find some wacky candidates from parties you've never heard of, radio-station hosts, D-list celebrities, porn stars, and so on. Who's going to bow out first?

THE WINNER GETS ....

WHO WON? ....

DATE ....

SPECIAL PROVISIONS ....

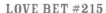

Predict the late shows' political jokes.

For instance, if the president falls down a flight of stairs, what will the jokes be?
Here's where you get to show off your sense of humor by predicting what the late
shows' writers are going to come up with. Tie the politician to one of that late night
host's favorite celebrity targets, and you're all set!

THE WINNER GETS	....
WHO WON?	....
DATE	....
SPECIAL PROVISIONS	....

Will your presidential team win the election?

You might have to wait until the next morning for the recount, or perhaps weeks for
the lawyers to decide, but the answer will come soon enough.

THE WINNER GETS	....
WHO WON?	....
DATE	....
SPECIAL PROVISIONS	....

LOVE BET #217

How long will it take them to recount the votes and make it official?

Make this bet to the day, such as three days, nine days, thirteen days, etc. The recount process can be very involved, with lawsuit after lawsuit piling up, if it's even remotely close. A concession may not come for weeks.

THE WINNER GETS	....
WHO WON?	....
DATE	....
SPECIAL PROVISIONS	....

LOVE BET #218

Name the winners of your local political elections.

Will the mayor be re-elected after he built up your town into a mega-shopping center? Will the judge candidate be elected after his son was found to have a DUI list a mile long? All the intrigue is in small town politics, since even small issues can be blown up into major crises—"He's been watering his lawn during the drought!" or "She has two vacation homes, so what does she know about being on the town council?!" It can be funny to follow the local columns and blogs.

THE WINNER GETS	....
WHO WON?	....
DATE	....
SPECIAL PROVISIONS	....

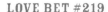

LOVE BET #219

What will be the next headline about the president's kids?

Underage drinking? An engagement? A bestselling book? Enrollment at Yale? Choose one media source, such as *People* magazine, to make this bet easier on you, and follow it closely for the next First Daughter or First Son mention.

THE WINNER GETS	....
WHO WON?	....
DATE	....
SPECIAL PROVISIONS	....

LOVE BET #220

The next celebrity couple to announce their engagement will be . . .

CELEBRITY NEWS

The media can't get enough of celebrity pairings and engagements, so when a ring comes into play, the story is splashed all over the covers of entertainment magazines and in breaking television news. They feed on predictions of who will be the next to marry, so take that nonstop celebrity coverage and turn it into your next fun bet.

THE WINNER GETS	....
WHO WON?	....
DATE	....
SPECIAL PROVISIONS	....

Who will be the next celebrity couple to break up?

Again, the gossip magazines and websites like TMZ.com are always filled with celebrity hookups and breakups—even going so far as to rank the best splits of all time (which is another bet you can make—who will be named the best breakup?). For now, narrow this bet to actual celebrities, such as those who appear in movies, and eliminate the faux celebs, like those who appear in reality shows.

THE WINNER GETS	....
WHO WON?	....
DATE	....
SPECIAL PROVISIONS	....

The next celebrity couple to have a baby will be . . .

You may follow the "baby-bump reports" in the media magazines and online, and you may know which celebrities donated all of their baby-shower gifts to charity. Make it fair to your partner by sharing a list of the almost-due celebs, and you'll each choose your next-to-deliver star.

THE WINNER GETS	....
WHO WON?	....
DATE	....
SPECIAL PROVISIONS	....

The next celebrity couple to adopt a baby will be . . .

Who's next? Angelina, Madonna, Meg? You can break this bet down into a 50-50 if you'd like: Choice 1, Angelina; Choice 2, Someone other than Angelina. And then check the reports in *People* and *Entertainment Weekly* to see who brought home a bundle of joy this week.

THE WINNER GETS	....
WHO WON?	....
DATE	....
SPECIAL PROVISIONS	....

Name the actor to be cast in the next big movie role.

Hollywood's been buzzing about the new blockbuster film franchise in the works, and every A-list actor is tap dancing to get the starring role. The entertainment magazines have run articles with the odds of which star or starlet will nab the role of a lifetime. If you're film buffs, you may want to set a Love Bet on this casting call.

THE WINNER GETS	....
WHO WON?	....
DATE	....
SPECIAL PROVISIONS	....

Who will be the top celebrity in the VH1 countdown you've been watching?

Don't you just love the VH1 countdown shows? They're perfect for a lazy night in, a snowy Saturday afternoon, even a day when you're both home sick with colds. Turn the hours invested in watching the countdown show into a bet, guessing which one of you can name the #1 spot. Or, which of your chosen celebrities is ranked higher than the other.

THE WINNER GETS	
WHO WON?	
DATE	
SPECIAL PROVISIONS	

LOVE BET #226

Name two of Barbara Walters's Most Fascinating People.

Every year, Barbara promotes her special by showing some of the winners ahead of time, but then she exhorts you to watch the show to see who's at the top of the list. Some of her choices may surprise you, so pick an odds-on favorite and a long shot from any area of entertainment, politics, and news headlines.

THE WINNER GETS	
WHO WON?	
DATE	
SPECIAL PROVISIONS	

Name the next *People* magazine's Sexiest Man Alive.

In the past, it's been Brad Pitt, George Clooney, and Matt Damon, among others. Who will top the list this year?

THE WINNER GETS	....
WHO WON?	....
DATE	....
SPECIAL PROVISIONS	....

Name the next *Maxim* magazine's Sexiest Woman Alive.

And again, you can twist this bet to have you both list your top ten.

THE WINNER GETS	....
WHO WON?	....
DATE	....
SPECIAL PROVISIONS	....

Name the next celebrity to pose for *Playboy*.

Every so often, a celebrity or faux-celebrity (meaning a reality show star who *thinks* she's a celebrity) agrees to shed clothing for cash. No matter how you feel about centerfolds ("It's art!" "It's trashy!"), you can turn this inevitability into a lover's bet that might get one of you to shed your own clothes.

THE WINNER GETS	....
WHO WON?	....
DATE	....
SPECIAL PROVISIONS	....

Name the next celebrity interview on *Oprah*.

It may seem like it's always John Travolta or Will Smith—two of Oprah's favorites—but she brings on authors and the casts of notable movies as well. So think ahead to movies coming out soon, and choose a celebrity from that list. Also possible: musical performers, since Oprah loves to throw a great concert in her studio.

THE WINNER GETS	....
WHO WON?	....
DATE	....
SPECIAL PROVISIONS	....

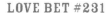

LOVE BET #231

Name the next celebrity to date your favorite professional athlete.

Can Tom Brady, Tony Romo, and Lance Armstrong possibly date some more celebrities? Choose your athlete stud and name the starlet he'll hook up with next.

THE WINNER GETS ....

WHO WON? ....

DATE ....

SPECIAL PROVISIONS ....

LOVE BET #232

Name the Razzie award winner for the year.

The Razzies are given to the worst film and the worst actors of the year. *Gigli* was one of those films in the past, for instance. So think about the box-office bombs this year, the truly awful performances, and get your bets in on who's going to take home the prizes.

THE WINNER GETS ....

WHO WON? ....

DATE ....

SPECIAL PROVISIONS ....

Name the winners of the MTV Movie awards.

Select your favorite categories and choose your winners.

THE WINNER GETS	....
WHO WON?	....
DATE	....
SPECIAL PROVISIONS	....

Name the next celebrity to get arrested, with his or her mug shot shown on television.

Or on TMZ.com, where mug shots get places of honor. As an added element to the bet, perhaps as a double-or-nothing, name what the charges are.

THE WINNER GETS	....
WHO WON?	....
DATE	....
SPECIAL PROVISIONS	....

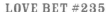

Name the next celebrity tell-all book.

If they have to be written, you might as well create a Love Bet on the next one to hit the bookstore shelves. It might be a steamy Hollywood tell-all or a here's-what-really-happened tome from a political insider. Whatever the topic, or how unbelievable the content, you win if you name the author correctly.

THE WINNER GETS	....
WHO WON?	....
DATE	....
SPECIAL PROVISIONS	....

Name the next celebrity to launch his or her own perfume or cologne.

Sarah Jessica Parker has her perfume, Marc Jacobs has his, and you can even smell like Donald Trump if you wanted to. When you look at perfume counters in department stores, you'll see some names that might surprise you. Think now about rising stars and starlets, and guess which one will add a perfume to his or her empire. For added fun, guess the name of that perfume.

THE WINNER GETS	....
WHO WON?	....
DATE	....
SPECIAL PROVISIONS	....

LOVE BET #237

Name the next celebrity to have a bare body part photographed by the paparazzi.

Somehow, celebutantes haven't learned how to get out of a car, and some are still not wearing panties. A strap slips off of a shoulder and there's another bare body part. We call them wardrobe malfunctions, but they're still skin shots. Who's going to be spotlighted next?

THE WINNER GETS	....
WHO WON?	....
DATE	....
SPECIAL PROVISIONS	....

LOVE BET #238

Name the next "star" of a celebrity sex tape.

True, some celebrities have no shame, and some of their chosen partners have no soul. When news of a new sex tape gets out, it seems that plenty of people want to take a peek. Even if you're not the voyeuristic types, and you'd never watch a tape like this, it's still a fun bet to guess which "star" wasn't smart enough to say "put the camera away" or "give me the tape."

THE WINNER GETS	....
WHO WON?	....
DATE	....
SPECIAL PROVISIONS	....

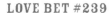

Name that cellulite!

Tabloids are always taking photos of celebrities' cottage-cheese thighs, so name the owner of those thighs the next time you're in line for groceries.

THE WINNER GETS	
WHO WON?	
DATE	
SPECIAL PROVISIONS	

Which celebrity will win the reality show he or she is now appearing in?

It might be a diet show, *The Surreal Life,* you name it. Who has the best odds of beating the other C- and D-listers?

THE WINNER GETS	
WHO WON?	
DATE	
SPECIAL PROVISIONS	

LOVE BET #241

Who was the other man/woman in a celebrity's breakup?

Tabloid reports speculate endlessly when a celebrity couple splits, but it often comes out later who the real home wrecker was—even if they deny it. Be careful with this bet if you're early in a relationship, since you don't want to seem like you revel in others' misfortune or that you don't take cheating seriously or that you have no empathy for the kids of that marriage. If you each have your suspicions and have discussed it, then it's okay to make a little wager on the outcome.

THE WINNER GETS	....
WHO WON?	....
DATE	....
SPECIAL PROVISIONS	....

LOVE BET #242

Name the next celebrity to launch his or her own clothing line.

Gwen Stefani has L.A.M.B.; Jennifer Lopez has her clothing line; as do Sarah Jessica Parker and others. Who's going to be the next fashion mogul?

THE WINNER GETS	....
WHO WON?	....
DATE	....
SPECIAL PROVISIONS	....

LOVE BET #243

Guess the next celebrity baby name.

This one can be tough, with celebrities getting so creative with their babies' names, so this is a fun one to discuss before you settle on a name for your favorite celebrity's baby.

THE WINNER GETS	....
WHO WON?	....
DATE	....
SPECIAL PROVISIONS	....

LOVE BET #244

Will the hardwood floor underneath that carpet need any repair work?

WORK ON THE HOUSE

Sometimes, you'll lift up a carpet and the hardwood floor will be perfect, only needing a polish. And sometimes, it has water damage or wood rot in some places. What condition is your floor going to be in?

THE WINNER GETS	....
WHO WON?	....
DATE	....
SPECIAL PROVISIONS	....

LOVE BET #245

Will the pest inspector find termites?

Carpenter ants? A bee infestation in the attic? The wait while the inspector pokes around can be nerve-racking, so turn this essential task into a wager that means good news either way.

THE WINNER GETS ....
WHO WON? ....
DATE ....
SPECIAL PROVISIONS ....

LOVE BET #246

Will the furniture fit through the door?

You may or may not have measured before ordering that couch, and sometimes furniture arrives in a different dimension than you were expecting. So when the delivery truck arrives, launch your bet about whether or not your beautiful new pieces are in the clear.

THE WINNER GETS ....
WHO WON? ....
DATE ....
SPECIAL PROVISIONS ....

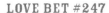

LOVE BET #247

Will the first attempt at hanging the cabinets be successful?

If you watch home remodeling shows, you know that hanging cabinets is a very tricky job. Everything has to be measured perfectly, every angle has to match, and your walls and ceiling have to be completely straight, which can be a challenge in an older house. So how is your attempt at hanging the cabinets going to go?

THE WINNER GETS	....
WHO WON?	....
DATE	....
SPECIAL PROVISIONS	....

LOVE BET #248

Will the project be completed by the deadline?

Both of you should be aware that many home remodeling and redecorating jobs take twice as long as you'd expect, so make sure you're both padding your guesses with some extra time.

THE WINNER GETS	....
WHO WON?	....
DATE	....
SPECIAL PROVISIONS	....

LOVE BET #249

Will the project come in under budget?

Ah, optimism. If this isn't your first big home project, you might know that the odds of coming in under budget are slim. So you might want to alter this bet to guessing the range of how far above budget you will be: $200 and under; $200–$500; $500–$1,000; or over $1,000, for instance. This bet takes trust, knowing that your partner is not going to buy a half dozen extra doorknobs just to push your expenses over that $200 budget. When both of you promise to keep expenses down, this bet can take the edge off of an oppressive budget and project.

THE WINNER GETS	....
WHO WON?	....
DATE	....
SPECIAL PROVISIONS	....

LOVE BET #250

Will the inspector show up on time?

If not, how late will he be? In the course of doing a major remodel, you'll become familiar with your town's rules about getting permits, having inspectors look over your work, and playing by the rules. Permits don't cost a lot; the real headaches come from waiting for an inspector who gives you a time range of "anywhere from 8:00 A.M. to noon," or later. So rather than raise your blood pressure waiting for him, get busy on another task and see what his arrival means for your bet.

THE WINNER GETS	....
WHO WON?	....
DATE	....
SPECIAL PROVISIONS	....

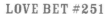

LOVE BET #251

Will the materials or tools you just bought for the project go on sale next week?

Check the weekend sales circulars to see if that jigsaw or that paint is now on sale for 30 percent off. This can be more than a bet; it can be a great motivator to get back to Home Depot or Lowe's to stock up on tools or paint.

THE WINNER GETS	....
WHO WON?	....
DATE	....
SPECIAL PROVISIONS	....

LOVE BET #252

How many times will you yell out an expletive while you're working on the project?

You might smack your finger with the hammer or drip some paint on the floor . . . whatever has gone wrong, you've spontaneously yelled out a bleeped-out word. Turn this into a bet that means the curser has to pay up whenever the R-rated language pops out.

THE WINNER GETS	....
WHO WON?	....
DATE	....
SPECIAL PROVISIONS	....

LOVE BET #253

What else will you find, besides leaves, in the gutter?

It could be a tennis ball from the neighborhood kids or it could be a rodent carcass. It's easier to face the surprises up there when you know you have a fun bet going.

THE WINNER GETS ....

WHO WON? ....

DATE ....

SPECIAL PROVISIONS ....

LOVE BET #254

Will you have to go back to the store to buy more tiles, paint, etc. after your initial-estimate shopping trip?

You did the math, you bought your supplies, but there's some essential that you're missing. It happens to professional contractors and decorators all the time, so don't let the stress get to you. Each time you have to stock up, turn this probable scenario into an okay-to-lose bet.

THE WINNER GETS ....

WHO WON? ....

DATE ....

SPECIAL PROVISIONS ....

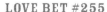

LOVE BET #255

Will the furniture be delivered on time?

A fun twist to this bet is that some companies deliver the furniture before their estimated delivery date. So it might be worth it to make this a before or after bet, rather than adding more stress by watching the calendar to gauge just how many days late the furniture is.

THE WINNER GETS ....

WHO WON? ....

DATE ....

SPECIAL PROVISIONS ....

LOVE BET #256

Which of your friends who offered to come and help will not show up?

Yes, you're betting that someone will let you down, but when you know it's just how they are, it's a little easier to take . . . especially when you make a great wager that allows you to win something from their no-show. Again, you're adding a positive spin to one of life's little bummers.

THE WINNER GETS ....

WHO WON? ....

DATE ....

SPECIAL PROVISIONS ....

LOVE BET #257

How many people will attend your first open house?

Do this one in a range, from one to five people, six to ten people, over ten people, etc. Bear in mind that your optimism is showing with this bet, so don't be the glass-half-empty type by guessing that no one will come. Remember, you're sharing Love Bets with your partner to show all the facets of how terrific you are, so be positive.

THE WINNER GETS	
WHO WON?	
DATE	
SPECIAL PROVISIONS	

LOVE BET #258

Today, the workman (plumber, contractor, etc.) will be wearing which color shirt?

If he's not in uniform, you might notice that he alternates between two or three shirts, or that he always has a beer-logo shirt on, or a sports-team logo shirt. Guess his wardrobe for the day, and cash in on your wager.

THE WINNER GETS	
WHO WON?	
DATE	
SPECIAL PROVISIONS	

Will you see a plumber's crack?

If you're not familiar with the term, a plumber's crack is seen when a laborer bends over in front of you, and you can see the top of his buttocks, including the "crack." Workers in ill-fitting jeans or workpants all across the country fall prey to this fashion faux-pas, to the amusement of those hiring them. As a caveat to this bet: This one has to be visually verified by you and your partner.

THE WINNER GETS	....
WHO WON?	....
DATE	....
SPECIAL PROVISIONS	....

Guess the cost of a major redecorating item purchase, such as a sofa, new bathtub, etc.

When you first start with a home remodel, or if this is your first home purchase, you will likely be way off on your guesses, but you'll get better as you gain more exposure in the world of home redo's. So making more and more price-guessing bets with your partner shows your progress and your growing smarts in this realm. Whoever's closest to the actual price wins.

THE WINNER GETS	....
WHO WON?	....
DATE	....
SPECIAL PROVISIONS	....

LOVE BET #261

Will you pass inspection on the first try?

Again, cut down the tension of the wait by turning this essential report into a wager. And, again, think about staying positive for this one!

THE WINNER GETS	....
WHO WON?	....
DATE	....
SPECIAL PROVISIONS	....

LOVE BET #262

Which word will (Relative/Friend) use when he/she sees the wall color for the first time?

You know your mother/sister/friend/father/brother. You know if the reaction is going to be positive and complimentary or if it's going to be sour grapes and unnecessarily critical. So each of you can choose three words that this person might use to comment on the wall colors and then listen for the first reaction. It could be, "Wow, that's bright!" or "That's so *earthy*" or "relaxing" or "a little much." Some couples who know the mother is jealous about the new partner's presence in the house can have some fun with her certain insult by guessing the passive-aggressive swipe.

THE WINNER GETS	....
WHO WON?	....
DATE	....
SPECIAL PROVISIONS	....

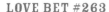

How many days will it take to get an offer on your house?

Be positive! It's the best way to attract an offer and impress your partner with your belief in your work on the place.

THE WINNER GETS	....
WHO WON?	....
DATE	....
SPECIAL PROVISIONS	....

What will be under that paneling?

Will it be plain wallboard or 1970s wallpaper with geometric patterns? Guess the pattern and the color for the big reveal.

THE WINNER GETS	....
WHO WON?	....
DATE	....
SPECIAL PROVISIONS	....

What will the realtor's market-value price be?

You know what you would like to price the house at, but what does the expert have to say? After all of your hard work, how much have you raised the property's value? Form your wager in ranges, such as Above $X or Below $X.

THE WINNER GETS	....
WHO WON?	....
DATE	....
SPECIAL PROVISIONS	....

What will the first offer be?

Since few people offer the asking price right away, pick out a fair number under your asking price and claim your price ranges in $20,000 increments. Some couples make charts in those $20,000 increments, and they write their names in the blocks they choose. If the offer hits within your block, you win.

THE WINNER GETS	....
WHO WON?	....
DATE	....
SPECIAL PROVISIONS	....

LOVE BET #267

Will there be a bidding war for your house?

It's wonderful to imagine several buyers bidding against each other and driving the price up because they love your house and property so much. Regardless of what the real estate market is like, these types of bidding wars take place all the time, all over the country. Your home might be the next in demand.

THE WINNER GETS	....
WHO WON?	....
DATE	....
SPECIAL PROVISIONS	....

LOVE BET #268

Will the buyer's financing come through?

It can be a white-knuckler until you get the call that all is clear, the buyer's financing has been approved, and your closing date is set.

THE WINNER GETS	....
WHO WON?	....
DATE	....
SPECIAL PROVISIONS	....

LOVE BET #269

Will it rain on our moving day?

When you're planning to move, you'll undoubtedly keep a close eye on the weather predictions. Is it going to be a scorching hot day? If rain is in the forecast, you may panic over how to protect your good furniture which will have to be carried out to the truck. You may worry about the moving crew's muddy boots tracking through the house. Since you can't predict the weather, you can take the edge off your worries by turning this into a bet. And be sure to specify what qualifies as "rain". A two-minute sprinkle on the morning of the move? Or a downpour?

THE WINNER GETS	....
WHO WON?	....
DATE	....
SPECIAL PROVISIONS	....

LOVE BET #270

How many repetitions will be completed when naked pull-ups guy (or any exhibitionist exerciser) works out?

WHAT THE NEIGHBORS WILL DO

If you have an exhibitionist neighbor living across the way from you, you might have caught a glimpse of Mr. Awesome doing naked pull-ups in front of his window. Especially in buildings with a narrow alley between them, you can often see your neighbors doing all sorts of things. Not everyone closes the shades. If you have a "look at me" neighbor, turn him into a source of bets rather than getting offended.

THE WINNER GETS	....
WHO WON?	....
DATE	....
SPECIAL PROVISIONS	....

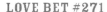

And of course, the kinky woman across the street— what's the show this evening? A male visitor? A new S&M outfit?

It's not always naked pull-ups or weightlifting going on across the street. Some neighbors get a kinky thrill out of leaving the shades open and risking "being seen" during their seductions. It gives them that "sex in public" rush without risking being arrested in the park. If you have *that* neighbor, her conquests can be a source of thrills for you when you make your own racy bets.

THE WINNER GETS	....
WHO WON?	....
DATE	....
SPECIAL PROVISIONS	....

Will the neighbor's teenage daughter's goodnight kiss be in the car, at the door, or will you see some more intense action within the car?

The neighbor's daughter comes home from dates at her midnight curfew pretty much like clockwork. It's not that you're spying on the neighbors; the loud music coming from the car gets everyone's attention, so you can't help but notice.

THE WINNER GETS	....
WHO WON?	....
DATE	....
SPECIAL PROVISIONS	....

LOVE BET #273

Will the neighbors leave the shades up in their bathroom again?

Some neighbors don't quite understand that even though they're on the second floor of their home, an open window still allows a view. So if your hairy-backed neighbor can be seen getting into his shower, or (ahem) sitting down for some reading time, that's a bet ready to be won by you.

THE WINNER GETS	....
WHO WON?	....
DATE	....
SPECIAL PROVISIONS	....

LOVE BET #274

Will you hear the neighbor's bed squeaking tonight?

You can hear everything that your upstairs neighbor does, including when he or she has . . . company. Notes haven't worked, and you don't make eye contact in the elevator anymore. Since the bed squeaking is going to continue, you might as well cash in on the action they're getting.

THE WINNER GETS	....
WHO WON?	....
DATE	....
SPECIAL PROVISIONS	....

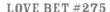

Name that smell.

What is the neighbor cooking tonight? Or is that incense he's burning? If your neighbor regularly has fantastic scents coming from his place, don't be afraid to knock on the door to give a compliment and ask for a recipe.

THE WINNER GETS	....
WHO WON?	....
DATE	....
SPECIAL PROVISIONS	....

Will the neighbor add a certain type of holiday décor to their house this year?

For instance, you could name the color of the lights they put up, guess which kind of giant inflatable character they'll buy this year to add to their collection, and so on.

THE WINNER GETS	....
WHO WON?	....
DATE	....
SPECIAL PROVISIONS	....

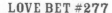

LOVE BET #277

Will the neighbors mow their overgrown lawn before Saturday?

They're the only ones in the neighborhood who don't have a landscaping service, and they always seem to let their lawn get out of control. Have some fun with their slacking by betting on whether or not they'll take care of it this weekend.

THE WINNER GETS ....
WHO WON? ....
DATE ....
SPECIAL PROVISIONS ....

LOVE BET #278

What will be the next thing the neighbors come over to borrow?

A few eggs? A hand mixer? A garden tool? If you have mooch neighbors who save money by using your stuff, laugh off their habits by turning them into some fun wagers of your own.

THE WINNER GETS ....
WHO WON? ....
DATE ....
SPECIAL PROVISIONS ....

LOVE BET #279

What color will they paint their house?

You can see that they're getting ready to paint their house or change their siding, so make your bets on which color they'll go with. Will they stick with the plain beige they've always had, or will they switch to a sunnier yellow with green shutters? Is this the year their house will look more modern?

THE WINNER GETS	....
WHO WON?	....
DATE	....
SPECIAL PROVISIONS	....

LOVE BET #280

Will the neighbors invite you to their child's wedding?

You've socialized with them often, and perhaps you've been invited to their child's graduation parties in the past. But when it comes to something big like a wedding, will you be on the guest list?

THE WINNER GETS	....
WHO WON?	....
DATE	....
SPECIAL PROVISIONS	....

Will the neighbor's kid's party get busted up by the police?

The parents are away, and the party is in full swing. Cars line the street, drunk kids are making out on the lawn, the music's loud, and you can hear things breaking. Will the lights and sirens of police cars be next on the scene?

THE WINNER GETS	....
WHO WON?	....
DATE	....
SPECIAL PROVISIONS	....

Will the neighbors put a stork sign on the lawn when they have their baby?

Or, will the new baby décor be pink, blue, or both, as in the case of twins?

THE WINNER GETS	....
WHO WON?	....
DATE	....
SPECIAL PROVISIONS	....

Will the neighbors sell their house before winter?

It's a gorgeous house, and you have no idea why it's still on the market after all this time. You know that the neighbors are anxious to sell—maybe they're building a new place in the mountains—so for their sake, you hope an offer comes in soon. So this Love Bet is made out of love for them, and you can weave the wager into something in the giving realm.

THE WINNER GETS	....
WHO WON?	....
DATE	....
SPECIAL PROVISIONS	....

What will be the first delivery to the new neighbors' house?

They've moved in, and you've brought them a basket of brownies to welcome them. As they're prepping their new home, what's going to be the first big purchase to come out of that furniture truck? A new bed? A new sofa? A flat-screen television? Keep an ear out for the rumble of a delivery truck and steal a peak at their new big buy.

THE WINNER GETS	....
WHO WON?	....
DATE	....
SPECIAL PROVISIONS	....

Will the new neighbors have a pet? If so, what will it be?

A Golden Retriever? Pekingese pups? A fat cat in the window scowling at everyone? It could be great to connect with the new neighbors over a shared love of pets.

THE WINNER GETS ....

WHO WON? ....

DATE ....

SPECIAL PROVISIONS ....

Predict when renting neighbors will move out.

They're cranky. They're loud. They're messy. They don't make an effort to get to know the neighbors. They speed through the residential areas. They don't say hello. You can't wait for them to move out so that better people can move in. When will they choose not to renew their lease?

THE WINNER GETS ....

WHO WON? ....

DATE ....

SPECIAL PROVISIONS ....

YOUR PERSONAL GOALS

LOVE BET #287

You will go a week without smoking/ drinking/eating junk food, etc.

It's tough to break a bad habit, but in this challenge, you're using the fun of the bet to motivate you. Your partner is not betting against you as a form of sabotage. It's a form of positive reinforcement, and he or she is really hoping you win this one! So choose your bad habit and put it on the betting block.

THE WINNER GETS ....

WHO WON? ....

DATE ....

SPECIAL PROVISIONS ....

LOVE BET #288

You will go two weeks without smoking/drinking/ eating junk food, etc.

Your partner is so proud of you, and you're both raising the bar to show how strong you are. Your partner is saying, "I know you can do it, even as you struggle with each craving and temptation. I have faith in you."

THE WINNER GETS ....

WHO WON? ....

DATE ....

SPECIAL PROVISIONS ....

You will go a month without smoking/drinking/eating junk food, etc.

They say it takes twenty-one days to break a habit, so you've conquered an addiction or bad habit! This is something to celebrate!

THE WINNER GETS	....
WHO WON?	....
DATE	....
SPECIAL PROVISIONS	....

You will give up a bad relationship with a troubled friend who drains your energy, which means no taking his/her calls, no agreeing to go out, no sliding backwards, no doubting yourself, and no doing favors just to be liked.

You don't need a friend like that, and I know you know that. So the wager is no contact with this toxic user for two weeks.

THE WINNER GETS	....
WHO WON?	....
DATE	....
SPECIAL PROVISIONS	....

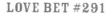

You'll go to the doctor for a full checkup or a mammogram.

If either of you has a too-packed schedule and can't seem to find time for essential self-care, this Love Bet comes from a place of deep caring for the other. You're providing positive reinforcement for making time to see the doctor or get the test.

THE WINNER GETS ....

WHO WON? ....

DATE ....

SPECIAL PROVISIONS ....

You will go to the gym three times a week.

Make the frequency realistic, not seven days a week. And let your partner decide which time of day works best: mornings or evenings. It takes a few tries to find the pattern that's going to stick, so support your partner's efforts with a great Love Bet, and join in so that you can both live a long, healthy, and happy life together. If your partner doesn't fulfill the three-times-a-week commitment, you get the wager for now. Then you can propose the same bet in a different form later on.

THE WINNER GETS ....

WHO WON? ....

DATE ....

SPECIAL PROVISIONS ....

You will join me in trying a new sport.

It might be tennis or golf or biking, whatever interests you both.

THE WINNER GETS	....
WHO WON?	....
DATE	....
SPECIAL PROVISIONS	....

You will begin a program of yoga, meditation, tai chi, or other relaxation program and maintain it for a month.

This one works best if you currently practice this relaxation program and wish to share it with your partner. Not that you should preach; it's just a shared activity that could keep you close.

THE WINNER GETS	....
WHO WON?	....
DATE	....
SPECIAL PROVISIONS	....

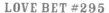

LOVE BET #295

You'll learn more about healthier nutrition and healthier cooking.

If your partner has expressed an interest in living a green lifestyle, eating locally grown foods, or going vegan, support this healthy outlook by making a bet about attending a healthy cooking class at the local education center or organic supermarket. If your partner follows through, you'll be happy to pay up.

THE WINNER GETS ....

WHO WON? ....

DATE ....

SPECIAL PROVISIONS ....

LOVE BET #296

You will complete your resume by Saturday.

It's not the most fun task ever, so you or your partner may need a Love Bet as motivation to get it done. The helpful partner can show that they want the resume maker to win by bringing them a cup of hot cocoa or a snack, reading the resume over for any typos, and sharing a supply of resume paper.

THE WINNER GETS ....

WHO WON? ....

DATE ....

SPECIAL PROVISIONS ....

LOVE BET #297

You will send your resume out by next Saturday.

Doubt can be paralyzing, so the resume writer may stall at the point of sending it out and taking a risk. So, again, build motivation with a great Love Bet.

THE WINNER GETS	....
WHO WON?	....
DATE	....
SPECIAL PROVISIONS	....

LOVE BET #298

By next week you will resign from two of your volunteer activities to have more time to yourself.

This is a tough one for people pleasers to even consider, since the group needs them. But it's essential for the overloaded partner to put himself or herself above the committee. He or she can be a leader in your home instead. So build motivation with a bet.

THE WINNER GETS	....
WHO WON?	....
DATE	....
SPECIAL PROVISIONS	....

LOVE BET #299

You will complete the organizing process you've been wanting to do in the garage, home office, kids' rooms, etc. by next month.

Give your partner a full thirty days to figure out a game plan, get the supplies needed, and embark on the task. And offer your services as a helper—it's not fair to expect him or her to tackle this big job alone. The thirty-day deadline is a realistic motivator.

THE WINNER GETS	
WHO WON?	
DATE	
SPECIAL PROVISIONS	

LOVE BET #300

We will renew our wedding vows, either as a big wedding do-over or just the two of us repeating our vows to one another in private.

Our relationship is so important to me that I'd love to make it a regular practice for us to express our appreciation of one another. It's great for the kids to see what a real marriage looks like, too.

THE WINNER GETS	
WHO WON?	
DATE	
SPECIAL PROVISIONS	

THE WAGERS

So what else would you like to win? A full-body massage in a room filled with candles and soft music? A gourmet dinner by the fireplace, each tender morsel hand-fed to you? A slow dance under the stars? A trip to Mexico? A love letter written by your sweetheart? Or maybe you just want the front lawn landscaped . . . finally!

Your definition of the perfect prize is completely up to you, what you feel you want, need, and would enjoy the most. You've read a few wagers in this book already; now, we're giving you even more! In this section, you'll find a vast collection of ideas broken down into different categories meant to inspire you both. You can flip through these to select the reward you most want for your win, choosing a different one each time, or just cashing in on that full-body massage (or that striptease) over and over again.

As a reminder, no wager should ever make your partner feel uncomfortable or resentful. That works against the whole point of this book, which is to bring you closer and more connected to one another. Your partner gets a clear message of what it is that you consider romantic, racy, or just realistic.

Go through now and star or circle the wagers you love the most. Cross off the ones you'd never want in a million years or those that are outside your comfort zone. Have your partner do the same. How else would you ever know that he really wants to see you wash his car while wearing his old high school football jersey and a tight pair of shorts? That kind of thing doesn't usually come up over breakfast.

The wagers are broken down into tame, romantic, and racy, and you'll also find some additional categories at the end if the occasion doesn't call for a romantic or sexy wager. If you're betting on your kid's softball game, for instance, it would be just wrong to wager for something racy. That might be a bet to negotiate an afternoon where he takes the kids (or your sister's kids that you're watching for the weekend) and sends you off to a day spa for a mani/pedi.

If you work this book right, you might (or will) turn your relationship into a living example of appreciation, laughter, and reminding each other of the sensual and thoughtful people you are. And most of all, you get to play together. This entire book is about taking the everyday events of your life and adding novelty to them, turning the present into a present that gives back again and again when you read back over how much fun you've had together since starting the shared activity of romantic wagers and couples' bets.

Ready for some inspiration? The wagers are ready for you to select.

TAME

You won't find any stripteases here! These wagers are tame by nature, which might suit the stage of your relationship way better than anything romantic or racy. And of course, even if you are in a romantic and racy relationship or marriage, these rewards can be perfect within your repertoire of regular bets with one another.

FOOD AND MEALS

☐ I'll make your favorite dinner. You choose the menu and I'll serve it to you here at home in the dining room.

☐ I'll make your favorite dinner. You choose the menu and I'll serve it to you al fresco, out on the deck or in the yard.

☐ I'll make dinner every night this week.

☐ I'll do all the cooking for our upcoming family event (holiday, kid's party, relative's visit, etc.).

☐ I'll make all the snacks for our upcoming movie or game night with friends.

☐ I'll make the very first meal I ever prepared for you at the start of our relationship.

☐ I'll take you to the restaurant of your choice.

- [ ] I'll have your favorite dinner delivered to us at home.

- [ ] I'll prepare a picnic for you, served at your choice of park or in the backyard, complete with red-checked blanket and Frisbee.

- [ ] I'll prepare breakfast for you, served at the kitchen table on the good china.

- [ ] I'll prepare breakfast for you, served in bed.

- [ ] I'll take you to a five-star brunch at a top hotel or restaurant.

- [ ] I'll take you for a breakfast out at the beach or park.

- [ ] I'll bring you breakfast at work.

- [ ] I'll take you out for lunch at your favorite restaurant.

- [ ] I'll take you out for lunch at a surprise locale that I choose.

- [ ] I'll take you—and the kids and your parents—out for lunch.

- [ ] I'll bring you lunch at work.

- [ ] I'll have a surprise lunch delivered to you at work.

- [ ] I'll bake you your favorite treat.

- [ ] I'll make or get you your favorite healthy treat (such as fruit salad, tropical fruits, fruit smoothies, etc.).

- [ ] I'll get you three bags of your favorite candies (M&Ms, jelly beans, etc.).

- [ ] I'll have M&Ms personalized for you. (Visit *www.mms.com* to see how you can custom create your own bags of colored M&Ms and personalize the messages and photos on them.)

- [ ] I'll pick up your favorite chocolates or truffles.

- [ ] I'll set up an ice cream sundae bar for you, featuring all your favorite flavors and toppings.

- ❏ I'll make you an ice cream float or milkshake.

- ❏ I'll take you out for ice cream.

- ❏ I'll take you and the kids out for ice cream.

- ❏ I'll take you out for dessert and coffee.

- ❏ I'll make you coffee every morning before work.

- ❏ I'll bring you coffee at work.

- ❏ I'll get you a fabulous bottle of wine.

- ❏ I'll get you a bottle of champagne.

- ❏ I'll serve you your favorite drink when you get home from work.

MASSAGE AND PAMPERING

- ❏ I'll give you a foot rub while we're watching television tonight.

- ❏ I'll give you a backrub while we're watching television tonight.

- ❏ I'll give you a hand massage with your choice of scented lotions that I will buy for you.

- ❏ I'll give you a ten-minute neck massage when you get home from work.

- ❏ I will run a bubble bath for you.

- ❏ I will get you a collection of bath salts and bubble baths.

- ❏ I will get you a gift certificate to your favorite pampering-product store or website (such as Bath and Body Works—see Resources).

- ❏ I will get you new fuzzy slippers.

- ☐ I will get you a comfy new spa robe.

- ☐ I will get you a gift certificate for a professional massage (choose from relaxing, sports, prenatal, etc.).

- ☐ I will get you a gift certificate for a reflexology session.

- ☐ I will get you a gift certificate for a manicure/pedicure.

- ☐ I will get you a gift certificate for a haircut at your favorite salon.

- ☐ I will get you a gift certificate for any treatment at your favorite salon.

- ☐ I will take the kids for an hour each night to give you relaxing alone time.

- ☐ I will get you the book you've been wanting to read during your relaxing alone time.

- ☐ I will get you a gift certificate for a yoga class.

- ☐ I will get your choice of relaxing music CDs.

- ☐ I will get you a basket of relaxing teas.

- ☐ I will get you a set of comfy new bath towels.

DATE NIGHT

I will take you:

- ☐ To the movies

- ☐ To a concert

- ☐ Out to dinner

- ☐ Out to lunch

- ☐ To your choice of theater production

- ☐ To a professional sporting event

- ☐ To a minor-league sporting event

- ☐ To a college sporting event
- ☐ To dinner with your friends
- ☐ To dinner with your family
- ☐ To a nightclub
- ☐ Bowling
- ☐ To a gallery opening
- ☐ To a festival
- ☐ Ice skating
- ☐ To a piano bar
- ☐ To look at houses decorated for the holidays
- ☐ To a scenic lookout
- ☐ To your class reunion

We'll stay in to:

- ☐ Watch your choice of movie, with a home-cooked dinner
- ☐ Watch your choice of movie, with takeout of your choice
- ☐ Watch a sporting event at home
- ☐ Watch a reality show at home
- ☐ Watch an awards show at home
- ☐ Have a game night featuring your choice of game
- ☐ Have dinner alone
- ☐ Watch our wedding video
- ☐ Just be alone, since I'm getting a sitter for the kids

A LITTLE GIFT

- ☐ Framed photos of you or the kids
- ☐ Restored family photos
- ☐ Family movies put onto DVD
- ☐ Music CD mix

- ☐ A DVD collection, whether movies or television series
- ☐ Your favorite author's new book
- ☐ An item for your collection

- A scrapbook

- Jewelry, such as a charm bracelet or locket

- A sporting item, such as a college-team T-shirt or a pro-team wristwatch

- Chocolates or candies

- A fun toy that reminds you of your childhood

- A gift certificate for your favorite home décor store or home fix-it store

- A replacement item for something that had been broken in the past, such as a vase

- Stationery or note cards with your name or monogram

BIG GIFTS

- A new handbag
- New shoes
- New golf club
- Tickets to a sporting event
- A round of golf at a great course

- A new jacket
- New shoes
- A digital camera upgrade
- Designer perfume or cologne
- "Pick out anything you want in this catalog"

HONEY DO

- [ ] Clean the entire house, including dusting and vacuuming.
- [ ] Clean a single room, including dusting and vacuuming.
- [ ] Clean out the garage.
- [ ] Clean out the attic.
- [ ] Create an organizing system for (fill in the room).
- [ ] Mow the lawn.
- [ ] Rake or vacuum the leaves.
- [ ] Do the mulching.
- [ ] Put in a new flower bed.
- [ ] Do the weeding.
- [ ] Pick the vegetables in the garden.
- [ ] Create a compost heap.
- [ ] Fix the leaky faucet.
- [ ] Paint a room.
- [ ] Put in hardwood floors.

- [ ] Put down new kitchen tiles.
- [ ] Clean out the gutters, carpets, curtains.
- [ ] Clean the sofa fabrics and pillows.
- [ ] Clean out the refrigerator.
- [ ] Clean out the freezer.
- [ ] Flip the mattresses.
- [ ] Organize the linen closet.
- [ ] Clean the kids' rooms.
- [ ] Take pets to the groomer's.
- [ ] Do the laundry for the week.
- [ ] Pick up the dry cleaning for the week.
- [ ] Clean the windows.
- [ ] Power wash the outside of the house.
- [ ] Organize a garage sale.

- [ ] Collect items to be donated to charity.
- [ ] Fix (fill in broken appliance).
- [ ] Have the cars cleaned and waxed.

- [ ] Get the car fixed (including new tires, changing the oil, etc.).
- [ ] Make an appointment with the professional we need to fix/install (insert item here).

SILLY STUFF

- [ ] Sing a childhood song.
- [ ] Sing at a karaoke bar.
- [ ] Wear mismatched clothes all day.
- [ ] Wear a joke tie to work.
- [ ] Wear a costume for the day.
- [ ] Agree to answer to a nickname that I make up for you.
- [ ] Do a celebrity impersonation.
- [ ] Dance to a song that I choose.
- [ ] Talk in an accent all day.
- [ ] Let the kids do your makeup for the day.

- [ ] Let the kids do your hair for the day.
- [ ] Let the kids pick out your outfit for the day.
- [ ] Dance in the rain.
- [ ] Sing out the car window during a family outing.
- [ ] Yell, "I love (your name)" out the window.
- [ ] Wear a silly slogan T-shirt all day.
- [ ] Apply a temporary tattoo where others can see it.
- [ ] Stand there while we shoot silly string at you.

- ❑ Stand there while we shove a pie in your face.

- ❑ Watch a comedy movie marathon with me.

- ❑ Do a skit with the kids.

- ❑ Re-enact your high school play, musical, skit, dance routine, cheerleader routine, sports warm up, or other performance.

- ❑ Dress in the archrival team's jersey while we watch the game (but not if you're going to the stadium, since at some stadiums this could put you in danger!).

- ❑ Paint your face in the team colors and we'll go to a sports bar or to the game.

- ❑ We will play videogames together.

- ❑ We will play the kids' board games together.

- ❑ We will go to a psychic together.

- ❑ We will finger paint together.

- ❑ You have to make me a sculpture out of clay or Play-Doh. Your choice of design.

- ❑ I get to take silly photos of you.

- ❑ I get to take a silly video of you doing that dance, singing that song, re-enacting that routine, etc.

- ❑ You have to call a friend and leave a completely silly message on their voice mail.

- ❑ You have to sing in the shower—loudly!

- ❑ You have to re-enact a movie scene chosen by me.

- ❑ You have to dance strangely at a family party or wedding.

- ❑ You'll let the kids choose what they want to see you do—hula hoop, jump on the trampoline, dress up in a tutu and have a tea party, etc.

ROMANTIC

N ow we're getting into the sweet offerings that make you feel loved and adored. You know what says romance to you—it might be flowers, it might just be the way you look at each other across the room. For your romantic bets, consider the following rewards:

FLOWERS AND CHOCOLATES

- ❒ I'll get you a bouquet of roses.
- ❒ I'll get you a bouquet of your favorite flowers.
- ❒ I'll get you a bouquet of flowers each week for a month.
- ❒ I'll put flowers in every room of the house.
- ❒ I'll fill the bedroom with flowers.
- ❒ I'll cover the bed with rose petals.
- ❒ I'll send flowers to you at work.
- ❒ I'll bring flowers to you at work.
- ❒ I'll put a single flower on your pillowcase each night for a week.
- ❒ I'll get you different-colored flowers every day of the week.
- ❒ I'll enroll you in the flower-of-the-month club.
- ❒ I'll get you a bouquet with one flower for every week we've been together (or month, if that's more appropriate).

- ☐ I'll get a bouquet of your birth-month flowers.

- ☐ I'll leave flowers on your car at work.

- ☐ I'll have flowers of your choice planted in the garden.

- ☐ I'll get you the same type of flower bouquet that I brought you when we got engaged.

- ☐ I'll put rose petals in your bathwater for you.

- ☐ I'll leave a path of rose petals from the front door to our bedroom.

- ☐ I'll spell your name out on the bed with rose petals.

- ☐ I'll leave a message spelled out in rose petals for you as a surprise in the bedroom, kitchen, etc.

- ☐ I'll get you chocolates and truffles from your favorite chocolatier.

- ☐ I'll get you chocolate-covered strawberries . . . and feed them to you.

- ☐ I'll make you chocolate-covered berries or cookies dipped in dark, milk, or white chocolate.

- ☐ I'll make a romantic chocolate fondue with lots of fruits and cake squares for dipping.

- ☐ We'll have a midnight fondue party by the fireplace.

- ☐ We'll go to the chocolate shop and you can pick out anything you'd like.

- ☐ I'll hand feed you chocolates while you're in the bathtub.

- ☐ I'll hand feed you chocolates in bed.

- ☐ I'll get you a heart-shaped box of chocolates.

- ☐ I'll get you a theme shape of chocolate from the specialty chocolate shop.

- ❐ I'll make a CD mix of all of "our songs."

- ❐ I'll make a CD mix of romantic songs that remind me of you.

- ❐ I'll make a CD mix of your favorite songs from our wedding.

- ❐ I'll have a song dedicated to you on the radio.

- ❐ I'll print up the lyrics of "our song." (Visit *www.songlyrics .com* and *www.elyrics.net* to get the exact words of your song.)

- ❐ I'll print up the lyrics of a song that reminds me of you.

- ❐ I'll frame the lyrics to "our song."

- ❐ I'll get concert tickets to see our favorite romantic recording artist.

- ❐ I'll serenade you under the bedroom window.

- ❐ I'll serenade you in public.

- ❐ I'll write a song for you and perform it only for you.

- ❐ I'll write a song for you and perform it at your birthday party.

- ❐ I'll create a journal of the songs from our love story and the stories they remind me of.

- ❐ I'll send you one iTunes song link at work each day this week.

- ❐ I'll get you a new iPod and load it with songs from me.

- ❐ I'll create a DVD with photos and video of us, plus songs from our love story.

- ❐ I'll have a romantic song playing when you get home from work each night this week.

- ❐ I'll make you CD mixes for your commute, time at the gym, during your business trip, etc.

MASSAGE AND PAMPERING

❏ I'll give you a full-body massage, with romantic music playing, candles lit, and aromatherapy oil.

❏ I'll sign us up for a couple's massage at a day spa. (Check out *www.massagenvy.com* to find a great site near you!)

❏ I'll massage your feet as we listen to romantic music.

❏ I'll run a bath for us, with candles, soft music, bubble bath, and warm towels waiting for us afterwards.

SHOPPING AND GIFTS

❏ I'll get you a new framed photo of the two of us.

❏ I'll make an appointment with a photographer to take romantic photos of the two of us.

❏ I'll create a photo album filled with my favorite photos of us.

❏ I'll get you a three-stone pendant or jewelry to signify past, present, and future.

❏ I'll get you a journey pendant.

❏ I'll get you a piece of jewelry with our birthstones together.

❏ I'll get you a heart earrings and necklace set.

❏ I'll get you new cufflinks.

❏ I'll get you initial/monogram jewelry.

❏ I'll upgrade your engagement or wedding ring with a new ring jacket or a new anniversary band.

❏ I'll get you a personalized item engraved with the date we met, the date we got engaged, the date we got married, etc.

- [ ] I'll get us a bottle of wine or champagne to toast our relationship.

- [ ] I'll pay for a shopping spree at the flower shop.

- [ ] I'll get you a romantic negligee or silky robe.

- [ ] I'll get a new work by your favorite artist.

- [ ] I'll get you a surprise gift (make it something you know that he or she looked at in a store and passed up).

- [ ] I'll get us a cashmere blanket for cuddling.

- [ ] I'll get you a movie DVD (make it a surprise—the very first movie you saw on a date together, along with the ticket stub you saved from that date).

- [ ] I'll get you new cologne or perfume (add a romantic note about how much you love how your partner smells, or what this scent reminds you of).

- [ ] I'll get you an item to use at a later date (make it something that you'll use at your future wedding, such as toasting flutes or cake-cutting knives).

SENTIMENTAL

- [ ] I will show you all the items I saved from our earliest days of our relationship (ticket stubs, show programs, dried rose petals, letters and cards).

- [ ] I will show you the love poetry I wrote when I was younger.

- [ ] I will write you a love letter.

- [ ] I will get you a different store-bought greeting card, saying how much I love you, for every day of the week.

- [ ] I will paint your portrait or draw a portrait of you.

PHONE CALLS AND E-MAIL

❐ I'll make a romantic phone call to you at work.

❐ I will send you different romantic love quotes every day of the week. (Sign up for the Love Quote of the Day at *www.brainyquotes.com*.)

❐ I will send you a love letter via e-mail at work or while you're away on a business trip.

❐ I will call you every day during my business trips—first thing in the morning, so mine is the first voice you hear.

❐ I will call you every night during my business trips, so that mine is the last voice you hear.

❐ I'll send you an e-mail listing all the things I love about you.

GETAWAYS

❐ We'll go for a weekend at a bed and breakfast. (Visit *www .BnBFinder.com* to find gorgeous ones near you or at a vacation destination.)

❐ We'll go for a weekend at a hotel.

❐ We'll revisit our first-ever vacation spot and stay the weekend there.

❐ We'll go for an overnight stay in the nearest big city.

❐ We'll go for a weekend getaway at the shore.

❐ We'll go for a weekend getaway at a ski resort.

- [ ] We'll go for a surprise weekend getaway. I'll choose the location and let you know what to pack.

- [ ] We'll go for a week's vacation anywhere you want.

- [ ] We'll go back to our honeymoon resort for a second honeymoon weekend.

- [ ] We'll choose our favorite destination from *www.traveland leisure.com*'s World's Best survey, and we'll book a vacation there.

- [ ] We'll watch the Travel Channel to choose our next vacation getaway.

- [ ] I'll get you new luggage for our next romantic vacation.

RACY

I t's time to get sexy! Here's where you peel off the clothes, tempt each other's senses, and enjoy the passion between you in a whole new way. It really doesn't matter who "wins," since everyone's a winner when your wager is one of these!

WARDROBE

- ❏ I will get or wear your choice of any lingerie, with thigh highs, stilettos, garters, and anything else you choose out of a catalog.

- ❏ I will surprise you with my choice of lingerie for the evening.

- ❏ I will only wear stiletto boots . . . and a smile.

- ❏ I will let you slowly undress me.

- ❏ I will wear your choice of sexy costume, whether it's a nurse, bunny, pirate girl—you name it.

- ❏ I will show up for dinner reservations in a sexy black dress, with or without sexy lingerie on underneath.

- ❏ I will wear body paint instead of clothes, and you get to apply it.

- ❏ Three words: chocolate body paint.

- ❑ I will dress up as your fantasy celebrity and role play with you.

- ❑ I will wear pasties for you.

- ❑ I will put on my wedding gown, then take it off slowly for you.

- ❑ I will undress while you watch.

- ❑ I will wear a French maid outfit and clean your home office while you watch. Then we'll clear off the top of your desk.

- ❑ I'll wear nothing but one of your work shirts and high heels.

- ❑ I'll wear the suit you love and let you undress me.

STRIPTEASE

- ❑ I'll perform a striptease for you.

- ❑ I'll perform a striptease for you to the song of your choice.

- ❑ I'll perform a striptease for you wearing your choice of outfit.

- ❑ I'll give you a lap dance.

- ❑ You'll get a different striptease every night this week.

JUST ADD WATER

- ❑ We'll go hot-tubbing together tonight . . . no bathing suits allowed.

- ❑ We'll do the wet T-shirt thing in the backyard tonight—you get to pour the water on me.

- ❑ We'll take a shower together.

- ❑ We'll go hot-tubbing together tonight.

- ❑ We'll have sex in the backyard pool.

- [ ] We'll have sex in the backyard hot tub.

- [ ] I'll go down the slide naked in our backyard pool.

- [ ] I'll dive off the diving board naked in our backyard pool.

- [ ] We'll swim naked in the backyard pool.

- [ ] We'll go to a nude beach together.

- [ ] We'll have sex on the beach.

FOOD ORIENTED

- [ ] You'll get blindfolded and I'll feed you different types of food.

- [ ] You get to eat whipped cream off my body.

- [ ] You get to lick chocolate sauce off my body.

- [ ] You get to lick caramel off my body.

- [ ] You get to lick honey off my body.

- [ ] We'll do tequila body shots.

- [ ] We'll have a naked dinner in bed.

- [ ] We'll have a naked breakfast in bed.

- [ ] Choose three different types of food to incorporate into our lovemaking tonight.

THE WRITTEN WORD

- ❏ You'll write an X-rated letter to me.

- ❏ You'll read me an erotic story from a book.

- ❏ You'll write an erotic story about me and read it to me.

- ❏ I'll send you a sexy e-mail (but not at work!).

- ❏ You'll write sexy captions for photos of us.

- ❏ We'll take sexy Polaroids of each other and you'll write sexy captions for each picture.

- ❏ You'll write sexy descriptions of your favorite parts of my body.

- ❏ You'll write an erotic story about the first time we made love.

THE SPOKEN WORD

- ❏ You'll call me for phone sex, even if you're calling from the next room.

- ❏ You'll tell me all the reasons you want to have sex . . . right now!

- ❏ Without touching me at all, you'll tell me all the things you want to do to me.

- ❏ You'll use the same dialogue from an erotic movie that we watch together, and we'll act out the same scene.

RESOURCES

FLOWERS
1-800-Flowers: *www.800flowers.com*
FTD: *www.ftd.com*
Martha Stewart: *www.marthastewart.com*
Teleflora: *www.teleflora.com*

CHOCOLATES
Burdick Chocolates: *www.burdickchocolate.com*
Chocolate Lovers: *www.chocolatelovers.com*
Ghirardelli: *www.ghirardelli.com*
Godiva: *www.godiva.com*
Hershey's: *www.hersheys.com*
See's Candies: *www.sees.com*
Seroogys: *www.seroogys.com*
Z Chocolat: *www.zchocolat.com*
M&Ms: *www.mms.com*

MASSAGE ITEMS

Drugstore.com: *www.drugstore.com*
Gaiam: *www.gaiam.com*
Massage Products: *www.massageproducts.com*
Mountain Rose Herbs: *www.mountainroseherbs.com*
The Body Shop: *www.thebodyshop.com*

LINGERIE

Bare Necessities: *www.barenecessities.com*
Bloomingdales: *www.bloomingdales.com*
Frederick's of Hollywood: *www.fredericks.com*
Macy's: *www.macys.com*
Target: *www.target.com*
Victoria's Secret: *www.victoriassecret.com*

MUSIC

Amazon: *www.amazon.com*
Barnes and Noble: *www.bn.com*
eLyrics: *www.elyrics.net*
iTunes: *www.itunes.com*
SongLyrics.com: *www.songlyrics.com*

WINE AND CHAMPAGNE

Wine Basket: *www.winebasket.com*
Wine Spectator: *www.winespectator.com*

EDIBLES

Berries.com: *www.berries.com*
Cheryl & Company: *www.cherylandco.com*
Gourmet Food Mall: *www.gourmetfoodmall.com*
Harry & David: *www.harryanddavid.com*
Maine Lobster Direct: *www.mainelobsterdirect.com*
Mrs. Fields: *www.mrsfields.com*
Omaha Steaks: *www.omahasteaks.com*
The Popcorn Factory: *www.thepopcornfactory.com*

PHOTO FRAMES

Bed Bath & Beyond: *www.bedbathandbeyond.com*
Crate & Barrel: *www.crateandbarrel.com*
Kate Spade: *www.katespade.com*
Lenox: *www.lenox.com*
Macy's: *www.macys.com*
Photo Fiddle: *www.photofiddle.com*
Pier 1: *www.pier1.com*
Shutterfly: *www.shutterfly.com*
Snapfish: *www.snapfish.com*
Vera Wang: *www.verawang.com*

EXTRA WAGER SHEETS

LOVE BET: _____

THE WINNER GETS	....
WHO WON?	....
DATE	....
SPECIAL PROVISIONS	....

LOVE BET: _____

THE WINNER GETS	....
WHO WON?	....
DATE	....
SPECIAL PROVISIONS	....

LOVE BET: _____

THE WINNER GETS	....
WHO WON?	....
DATE	....
SPECIAL PROVISIONS	....

LOVE BET: _____

> THE WINNER GETS ....
> WHO WON? ....
> DATE ....
> SPECIAL PROVISIONS ....

LOVE BET: _____

> THE WINNER GETS ....
> WHO WON? ....
> DATE ....
> SPECIAL PROVISIONS ....

LOVE BET: _____

> THE WINNER GETS ....
> WHO WON? ....
> DATE ....
> SPECIAL PROVISIONS ....

LOVE BET: _____

THE WINNER GETS ....

WHO WON? ....

DATE ....

SPECIAL PROVISIONS ....

LOVE BET: _____

THE WINNER GETS ....

WHO WON? ....

DATE ....

SPECIAL PROVISIONS ....

LOVE BET: _____

THE WINNER GETS ....

WHO WON? ....

DATE ....

SPECIAL PROVISIONS ....

LOVE BET: _____

THE WINNER GETS ....
WHO WON? ....
DATE ....
SPECIAL PROVISIONS ....

LOVE BET: _____

THE WINNER GETS ....
WHO WON? ....
DATE ....
SPECIAL PROVISIONS ....

LOVE BET: _____

THE WINNER GETS ....
WHO WON? ....
DATE ....
SPECIAL PROVISIONS ....

LOVE BET: _____

THE WINNER GETS	....
WHO WON?	....
DATE	....
SPECIAL PROVISIONS	....

LOVE BET: _____

THE WINNER GETS	....
WHO WON?	....
DATE	....
SPECIAL PROVISIONS	....

LOVE BET: _____

THE WINNER GETS	....
WHO WON?	....
DATE	....
SPECIAL PROVISIONS	....

LOVE BET: _____

THE WINNER GETS ....

WHO WON? ....

DATE ....

SPECIAL PROVISIONS ....

LOVE BET: _____

THE WINNER GETS ....

WHO WON? ....

DATE ....

SPECIAL PROVISIONS ....

LOVE BET: _____

THE WINNER GETS ....

WHO WON? ....

DATE ....

SPECIAL PROVISIONS ....

ABOUT THE AUTHOR

Sharon Naylor has been named "The Foremost Wedding Author in the Country." She is the author of thirty-five wedding books and has appeared on *Good Morning America*, *The Morning Show with Mike & Juliet*, *Inside Edition*, *Get Married*, Lifetime, and many other national shows. She is the iVillage Weddings etiquette expert, and their featured blogger on stress-free wedding planning. She has been featured in *InStyle Weddings*, *Brides*, *Modern Bride*, *Elegant Bride*, *New Jersey Bride*, the *New York Times*, the *Wall Street Journal*, and on Martha Stewart Weddings Sirius Satellite Radio. The idea for this book came from her practice of making non-monetary bets with friends and family, and she has won dinners, massages, and several romantic weekends away. Those who "beat" her at the bets won lobster bisque, chocolate mousse, massages, and a car wash. She believes the couple who plays together stays together. She lives in Morristown, New Jersey with her husband.

Printed in the United States
By Bookmasters